The Eye Book

To my wife, Dee, and my Mum, Gwen

'... to see clearly is poetry, prophecy and religion all in one'
John Ruskin (1819–1900)

THE EYE BOOK

Eyes and eye problems explained

Ian Grierson

LIVERPOOL UNIVERSITY PRESS

First published 2000 by
LIVERPOOL UNIVERSITY PRESS
4 Cambridge Street
Liverpool, L69 7ZU

British Library Cataloguing-in-Publication Data
A British Library CIP record is available

ISBN 0–85323-755–7 *paperback*

Typeset by Carnegie Publishing, Chatsworth Rd, Lancaster
Printed and bound in the European Union by
Biddles Ltd, Guildford and King's Lynn

Contents

Colour plates 1–17 appear between pages 88 and 89

Acknowledgements

I would like to thank Mrs Mary Kelley for her secretarial help and Dr Penny Hogg for assistance, particularly with respect to the diagrams. Help provided by Ms Ruth Madges (Pharmacia and Upjohn) was greatly appreciated. The text was reviewed by a number of people and among these I would like to single out for special thanks Mr James McGalliard (Clinical Director, St Paul's Eye Unit, Liverpool), Dr Chris Wigham (Department of Optometry and Vision Sciences, Cardiff), Mrs Gail Stephenson (Head of Orthoptics, University of Liverpool) and Dr Alan Canter (General Practitioner, Litherland).

Preface

The Eye Book has been a challenge to write because it walks a tightrope between being informative in the manner of a textbook and providing a book that is simply an interesting read about eyes. I intended a balance of both, but if I have slipped, then it is towards general interest. After all, there are many prestigious textbooks on eye structure and function, and just as many again that are totally unintelligible to the general reader who wants to know a little more about the most precious sense of sight.

Textbooks tend to be about eye structure, vision, visual aids, eye complaints and so on, but they rarely attempt to cover more than a narrow remit in great detail. What I have tried to do is to soar through all of these and also to embrace several other areas including the different kinds of eye professionals, historical eye care, famous people who have coped with eye problems, eye make-up, eyes in society, and eyes in mythology and religion. Finally I end up with a discussion of the appalling tragedy that is world blindness and what may be developed in the future to combat the ever-growing problem of visual handicap in both the developed and the underdeveloped world.

At whom is this book aimed? At everyone who has glasses or needs glasses, anyone who has a relative with an eye complaint, and basically all of us, because just about everyone will need to visit an eye professional at some time in their life. The general practitioner may find some parts of value, and I hope that the book will be a useful introduction for a student who is considering a future in orthoptics or optometry or for a nurse who might specialize in eye care.

As the book is not just for health-care professionals, I have tried to keep technical and medical words to a minimum. Unfortunately, however, I have had to include some specialized terms because eye professionals use them in their day-to-day work, and also too often when they try to communicate with their patients and the general public. If you do find an unfamiliar word (many of which are in italics at their first use) please refer to the glossary at the end of the book.

Ian Grierson

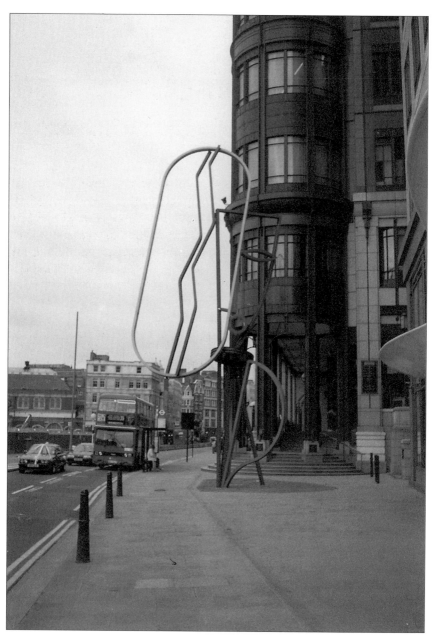

Frontispiece   The sculpture by Bruce McLean, called 'Eye-I', at Bishopsgate in London.

Chapter 1

Eye–I
The structure and function of the eye

Outside the Bishopsgate development near Liverpool Street Station in London is an abstract sculpture by Bruce McLean called 'Eye-I' (opposite). I don't know why Mr McLean chose this title but I misread it when I first saw it and wondered where 'Eye–2' might be! At least for me, the title of this dramatic, bold and colourful sculpture is an appropriate heading for this opening chapter. The chapter will deal with the structure and function of the human eye.

THE EXTERNAL EYE

The eye we see

Take a look at your eyes in the mirror and also refer to the first illustration (Figure 1.1). In painting classes, when drawing the face, we are told that the eyes come half-way down the head and that most of us when we first draw tend to make the error of positioning the eyes far too high.

The clear part at the front of the eye is the *cornea* and the white of the eye is the *sclera*. The coloured tissue behind the cornea and inside the eye is the *iris* and the dark opening in the centre is the *pupil*, which is wide in dim light and constricted in bright daylight. Not all of the iris circle can be seen when you look in the mirror because a segment is always covered by the open upper eyelid.

The eye we don't see

Pull back your eyelid gently and the hidden segment of iris can be seen. Look carefully and a transition region between the clear cornea and the white sclera may be evident. This is called the *limbus*. When the lid is pulled back, you will be able to see a large number of red blood vessels. These become even more obvious if there is dust or smoke in the eye, which then becomes red. Most of the vessels that can be seen are in a thin

1

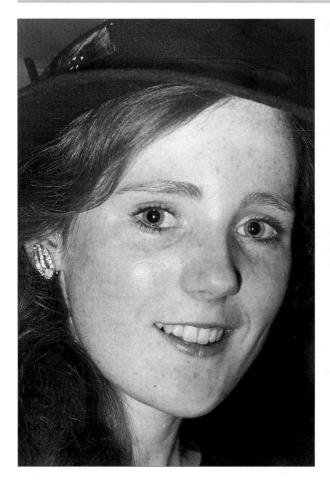

Figure 1.1 The eyes are nearly half-way down the head, as can be seen in this photograph of a young woman's face.

membrane of tissue on the surface of the sclera called the *conjunctiva*. The conjunctiva extends back and then over the inside of the upper lid. These blood vessels do not extend on to the clear cornea in a healthy eye. They are prevented from so doing by a number of biological and mechanical processes, because if vessels grew over the cornea, vision would be adversely affected.

On the surface of the conjunctiva are a host of cells called *goblet cells* and they, in conjunction with some small glands in the upper lid, release *mucus* and oils on to the surface of the eye. When you blink, the lid spreads the mucus and a watery fluid (tear fluid) from a structure called the *lacrimal gland* (see Plate 1) all over the cornea to keep it moist. The mucus has several functions, one being to act as a wetting agent so that the watery fluid spreads evenly as a fine film over the whole surface of the cornea. The oil cuts down the evaporation rate of the fluid spread over the mucus. A slow and steady production of fluid is important to lubricate the front of the cornea and to provide it with nutrients and oxygen. The tear fluid is also mildly sterilizing and contains substances which kill harmful bacteria. In some ways the tear water substitutes for the blood supply that the clear cornea, of necessity, does not have.

The blink of an eye

The fluid is continuously renewed and washed over the cornea with each blink, and it then drains away through a passageway called a duct which extends down into the nose (Plate 1). Tear fluid passes from the surface of the eye into the top of the duct through two fine channels. The openings of the channels are on either side of the *caruncle* (Plate 1), which you can feel as a small lump where the eyelids meet on either side of the nose. The caruncle, and the neighbouring tissue associated with it, is an evolutionary remnant of what was once a third lid. Some mammals still have a third lid for additional protection to the eye. It serves as a transparent shield when the other lids are open, allowing for instance, a camel to see safely during a sandstorm.

A minor condition in some babies occurs when the drainage duct is not open. In this situation the baby's eyes water excessively and the lacrimal sac must be popped by pressing in the region of the caruncle and the nose, thus putting pressure on the sac and forcing fluid down the drainage duct. Usually the problem causes more distress to the parents than to the baby and it rights itself in due course. As the baby grows, the drainage duct increases in diameter and usually opens up. If not, the opening can be cleared by a minor surgical manipulation.

Some older people, those with lid or orbital injury and patients with certain forms of illness such as rheumatoid arthritis can suffer from *dry eye*. This condition causes the eye to feel gritty and in severe cases the conjunctiva will become red and the sufferer will feel sharp pains in the eye. This can be due to insufficient tear fluid production resulting from atrophy of the lacrimal gland, but inadequate mucus production may also have a role. Without sufficient mucus the tear film is fragile and breaks up too soon, so the cornea is left with inadequate fluid cover. The usual remedy is to use one of the several artificial tear preparations available at the chemist's shop. If the condition is severe, surgical closure can be performed on the upper of the two fine channels by which tear fluid drains into the lacrimal sac. Because humans stand upright, the upper channel is used less frequently than it is in animals that walk on all fours with their heads down.

Tears for fears

Produced in excessive amounts, tear fluid may be too much for the tear ducts to cope with and so the surplus fluid will flood out on to the face. Such tears can be induced by a wide range of stimuli, for example, if you blink a lot, if you are emotionally upset, suffer a painful blow, come into contact with noxious chemicals (from onions* for example), have even a very minor injury to the eye, or are exposed to a cold wind, or if grit, a fly or some other foreign body makes contact with the eye or gets under a lid. This is one of the defence mechanisms that have evolved to protect the delicate eye from the hazards of an active life. So if a piece of grit gets under a lid and you can't see it to remove it with, say, the corner of a handkerchief, then the best thing is to blink rapidly and produce copious tears to wash out the offending object. Blinking is one of those processes which take place automatically but is also under conscious, voluntary control.

Floods of tears produced voluntarily or involuntarily are good protection but there are other forms. If an object comes close to our eyes, then we shut the lids immediately without even being aware of it. This is a protective reflex action which, for good reason, is extremely hard to overcome. There is a game played by children where a hand is waved closer and closer to someone's eyes until they close. The winner is the person who can resist reflex closure the longest and this is really difficult to do. Eyelashes have a role to play here because they set off the eye closure or blink reflex.

Our eyes are important to us so they are set deep into a bony socket and guarded by the nose, the cheek and particularly above by the brow. Together with the blink reflex and eye watering, there are simple mechanisms to protect the eyes from insults ranging from a dusty environment to being hit in the face by the branch of a tree. When a fighter is punched in the region of the eye in a boxing match, it is the brow which is cut, the cheeks which bruise and the nose which bleeds. The recessed eye is protected in the short term, although the continuous pounding can lead to problems such as retinal detachment (see later chapters for more information). Boxing referees will be on the lookout for unscrupulous fighters who may try sticking a thumb into their opponent's eye. A well-placed thumb will provoke the other protective mechanisms of blinking and watering, severely incapacitating the opponent.

Eye protection

Other primates, such as chimps, orang-utangs and some monkeys, have even

---

* Onions and garlic release volatile chemicals which react on the surface of the eye, to form sulphuric acid, in the case of onions.

more recessed eyes and deeper brow folds than humans. Vision is a very important sense for a tree-living animal and they must protect it while they move about, brushing into branches and foliage. However, there are many tree-living primates that have large protruding eyes, for example, lemurs and marmosets, and many living on the ground, such as baboons and gorillas, with pronounced eye recession and heavy brow ridges. It seems that animals with eyes at the front of their heads that are active during the daytime have heavy protection, whereas nocturnal animals (lemurs and the like) need big eyes to capture all the available light and they forgo the option of eye protection in favour of better sight in low illumination. Animals with eyes at the side of their heads frequently have little protection for them or even have eyes that stick out, such as is the case with the sheep, zebra, gazelle, deer or rabbit. These are usually grazers, for which eyesight is less important than a keen sense of smell. If smell lets them down, they need to have the widest possible field of view. They don't have to see clearly that it is a wolf, lion, fox or whatever; it is more important to detect movement or a blur as soon as possible without shifting their heads and then for them to run.

THE ORBIT AND EYEBALL

In the orbit

The bony housing for the eye is called the *orbit* and it is a pear-shaped structure into which the eyeball is recessed. Behind the eyeball is the narrowest part of the orbit and through here are openings to let in blood vessels and nerves to serve the ocular and orbital tissues. The principal opening is the *optic canal* through which the *optic nerve* (see later) passes on its way from the eye to the brain.

Extraocular muscles

The orbit contains fatty tissue to protect the eyeball (yet another defence mechanism) and a series of muscles which make the eye move. The muscles are connected to the outer coat of the eye in the manner shown in Figure 1.2 and are called *extraocular* (literally 'outside the eye') *muscles*. They belong to the muscle type known as *striped* (or striated) *muscle* (like the biceps in the arm) and are far more powerful and complex than the other type called *smooth muscle*. The muscles inside the eye are only of the smooth type. In all, there are six extraocular muscles for each eye, consisting of four rectus muscles and two oblique muscles. They are arranged in such a way that each is responsible for one of the major eye movements. Each muscle has a double name: the first for where it is located on the eyeball and the second for the family of muscles to which it belongs. These muscles are:

1 the superior rectus: extends backwards on top of the eyeball;

2 the inferior rectus: extends backwards underneath the eyeball;

3 the medial rectus: extends backwards at the side of the eyeball closest to the nose;

4 the lateral rectus: extends backwards at the side of the eyeball furthest from the nose;

5 the superior oblique: on the top of the eyeball extending over towards the nose and passing under the superior rectus; and

6 the inferior oblique: extends down under the eyeball towards the nose, passing over the inferior rectus.

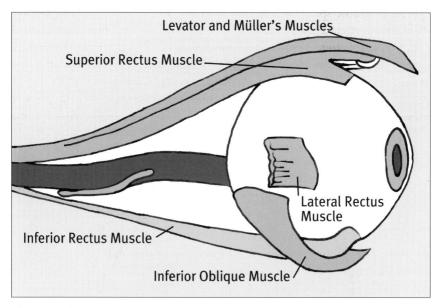

Figure 1.2 The white eyeball in side view showing the position of some extraocular muscles. (*Provided by Pharmacia & Upjohn, UK*)

The muscles control gaze and the contraction of these muscles leads to the movement of the eye in the appropriate direction. There are six basic movements of gaze. When you look to your right (3) you use the lateral rectus (4) of the right eye and the medial rectus of the left eye. Look to the left and it is the opposite way round: you use the right eye's medial rectus (3) and the left eye's lateral rectus (4). Up and right needs the superior rectus (1) of the right eye with the inferior oblique (6) of the left eye, whereas up and left gaze requires the inferior oblique (6) of the right eye and the superior rectus (1) of the left eye. Down and right is produced by contraction of the inferior rectus (2) on the right eye and the superior oblique (5) on the left eye. Down and left needs the superior oblique (5) of the right eye along with the inferior rectus (2) of the left eye. Looking straight ahead requires equal tone in all six muscles. Problems with the extraocular muscles that produce squinting and squints are dealt with in chapter 4.

Coats of the eyeball

The eyeball itself is made up of three different coats (Figure 1.3). The outer coat is fibrous and strong (cornea and sclera), the middle coat (*uvea*) is made up of blood vessels and provides the nutrition (see also Figure 1.7) and the inner coat is the nervous tissue (*retina*) which converts light into electrical impulses generating vision. The outer and middle coats are there primarily to protect or maintain the delicate inner coat. The human adult eyeball is almost spherical and varies quite a lot in size; it has an average diameter of around 24 mm, but can be as small as 20 mm in long-sighted people (*hypermetropes*) and as large as 29 mm in the short-sighted (*myopes*).

The shape of the eye is maintained by the pressure inside being a few millimetres of mercury higher than atmospheric pressure outside. On average the pressure difference is about 16 millimetres of mercury and the positive pressure is maintained by the circulation of a clear fluid called *aqueous*

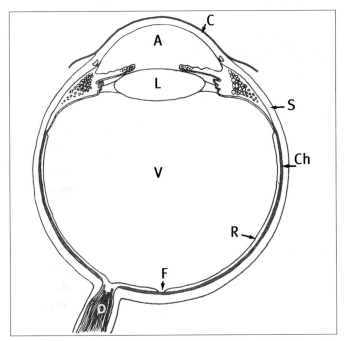

Figure 1.3 A diagram of the cross-section of the eye. The cornea (C), anterior chamber (A), lens (L), vitreous humour (V), sclera (S), choroid (Ch), retina (R), fovea of the macular region (F) and optic nerve (O) are indicated. (*Drawn by Alison Floyd, St Paul's Eye Unit, Liverpool*)

humour within the front chambers of the eye (see page 13). In terms of mechanics, the eye is constructed on a similar principle to a football, in that a tough but pliable outer coating remains firm owing to the pressure within. Such a sphere is light but robust, and has considerable strength without sacrificing either flexibility or elasticity.

THE FRONT OF THE EYE

Cornea

The structures of the front of the eye (Figure 1.3 and Plate 2) are primarily concerned with letting light into the eye, controlling the amount of light that reaches the back of the eye, focusing light on the retina, and establishing and maintaining the shape of the eye.

Let's look at the cornea. This is the window of the eye and as such it is transparent (Figure 1.3 and Plate 2). The cornea's main role is to bend light so that it can be focused on the retina; it is a more powerful lens than the lens itself which is more concerned with fine tuning. The bending of light rays in this way is called *refraction* in physics, so a lens is said to have a refractive power; the larger the refractive power, the stronger the lens (see also the section on glasses in chapter 3).

The outside surface of the cornea (Figure 1.4) is lined with several tiers of cells called epithelial cells. These rest on a basement membrane which in turn rests on a cell-free structure called *Bowman's membrane*. This *epithelium*

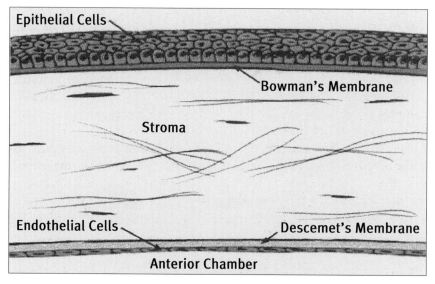

Figure 1.4 A diagram of the cornea in cross-section.
(*Provided by Pharmacia & Upjohn, UK*)

is continuous with the epithelium of the conjunctiva, the vascular membrane on the surface of the white coat called the sclera. The epithelial cells are a protective barrier and prevent foreign materials, bacteria, etc. from getting into the cornea. The cells also hold the mucus and oils of the tear film in place, and in turn gain nutrition from the film in the form of oxygen, minerals and glucose. A battery of sensory nerve endings are located here, resulting in this being a very sensitive tissue which is very painful if disturbed.

The bulk of the corneal substance is called the *stroma* (Figure 1.4), which is just a mass of extracellular material with a few cells called *fibroblasts* embedded in it. Fibroblasts are the constituent cell of connective tissue (gristle) and the stroma is a modified connective tissue. Like most connective tissue, the stroma consists of collagen fibres arranged in bundles and glued together with a complex mix of molecules which can be called ground substance. Unlike most connective tissue, the stroma has neither elastic fibres nor blood vessels; both of these are present in the adjacent sclera.

In the deepest part of the cornea the collagen fibres do not form bundles; this is called *Descemet's membrane*. A very thin basement membrane separates Descemet's from a single layer of endothelial cells. Basement membranes are so thin that they are hard to see even under an electron microscope, but they are essential in linking cell layers to connective tissue. Under the scanning electron microscope the cells of the endothelium form a honey-comb-like pattern (Figure 1.5). They are also very flat and that contributes to their transparency. This leads to the question: why is the cornea clear?

Scientists don't really know the reason for the cornea's transparency, but there are many theories. It is certainly the case that the collagen bundles in the stroma of the cornea form a very regular array, unlike in the sclera and other connective tissues where the arrangement of collagen bundles is very disorganized. The absence of blood vessels is very important, as is the lack of elastic tissue. In addition, the ground substance and the collagen have very similar refractive indices and these are maintained by the endo-thelium continuously pumping water out of the stroma.

The refraction of the cornea depends partly on how curved it is, but also on the difference in refractive index between the outside air and the cornea itself. You might liken this to the way that the water bends light when you look into a stream so that a fish that appears to be immediately under your net is actually off to one side.

Iris

The *iris* (see Plates 1–3, Figures 1.3 and 1.6) is the eye's shutter because its main function is to control the amount of light reaching the interior by altering the size of the hole in the middle called the *pupil.* The structure

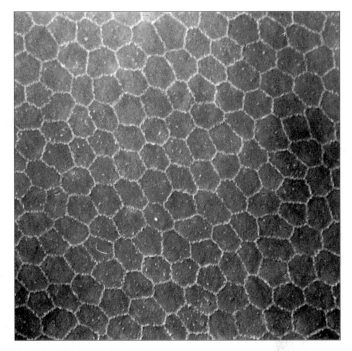

Figure 1.5   The flat mosaic of the corneal endothelium under the electron microscope.

of the iris in cross-section can be seen in Figures 1.3, 1.6 and Plate 3. It consists of a double layer of epithelial cells on the rear surface with a very loose connective tissue stroma in front. The stroma is quite different from that in the cornea: here there is much less collagen and the tissue is full of blood vessels. There are many more cells in this stroma; most prominent among them are fibroblasts, the principal cell of connective tissues, and *melanocytes*. Full of dark granules called melanin, melanocytes are responsible for pigmentation. In the skin they cause sun tan, and different quantities of melanin in hairs result in the different hair colours.

The epithelium consists of two layers of cells which also contain melanin granules, with these being particularly dense in the outermost layer (Plate 3). The two epithelial layers are quite different in appearance: the outer layer is made up of fat cuboidal cells, whereas the cells of the inner have a plump base and a long spindly head that links up with the heads of all the other cells in this region and extends down the iris towards the pupil rim. In fact the inner epithelial layer forms a primitive smooth muscle called the *dilator muscle*.

Remember, inside the eye all muscles are of the simple smooth type and there is a second smooth muscle in the iris called the *sphincter muscle*. The

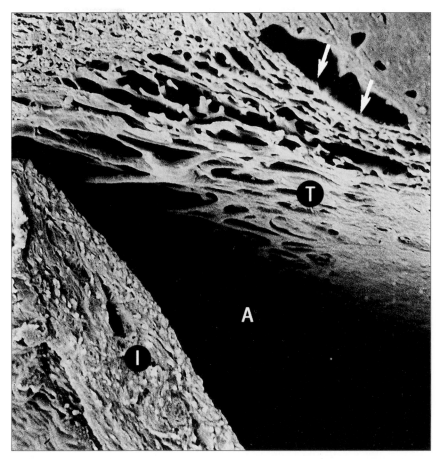

Figure 1.6 A view from the electron microscope of the outflow system showing the trabecular meshwork (T) and Schlemm's canal (arrow) that drain aqueous humour from the anterior chamber (A) out of the eye. Some iris (I) also can be seen.

dilator muscle peters out shortly before it reaches the pupil and this area is occupied by the sphincter. The sphincter is higher up in the stroma and extends as a circular sheet around the pupil, forming a muscular band less than a millimetre wide. The muscle fibre direction is at 90° to the dilator so that in cross-section it looks like a thin finger (Plate 3). The two muscle systems work automatically to cause the pupil to widen (dilate) in the dark or reduce (constrict) in bright light. This action is generally known as the light reflex.

The iris is a delicate mobile diaphragm (such as you find in a camera) acting to allow the greatest amount of light to reach the retina in gloomy conditions and to severely restrict the light entry in sunshine. The largest pupil diameter (see Figure 1.1) is around 8 mm and the smallest is only

1.5 mm. If we think again in terms of a camera, the focal length of the eye is about 20 mm, so pupil constriction between the two extremes is equivalent to going down in f stops from f13 to f2.5. For those of us who are not camera enthusiasts, this is around a 30-fold decrease in light let into the back of the eye.

Change in pupil size is necessary so that useful vision is available over the widest range of luminance. In the dusk we need all the light we can get to see our way, whereas excessive lighting conditions make vision (or *visual acuity*) difficult and can be overcome by a constricted pupil. Nocturnal animals have a greater problem than humans in bright sunlight and some have developed an oval pupil. The oval aperture of a cat's iris can close down to a slit and this is seemingly a more effective means of restricting light entry than our round pupil (see Plate 7).

There is another advantage to having a variable pupil and that is in *depth perception*. When the eye focuses on distant objects, depth of focus is not a problem so the pupil can be large. On the other hand, close-up objects have a small depth of focus and our view of them can be helped considerably by reducing pupil size. A small pupil lets through a narrow beam of light which in turn increases the depth of focus of our optical system. The cornea, like many lenses, is not optically perfect but is at its best in the centre; a narrowed pupil will therefore minimize any optical defects. In the dark these corneal defects are unimportant, but in daylight, when form is a significant part of vision, a reduced pupil is of optical benefit.

Strangely for such an important social and cosmetic feature, eye colour and the reason for its variations are still poorly understood. It is not for want of interest in the subject, yet mysteries remain despite the efforts of scientists for hundreds of years. The colour of the iris seems to depend on the light entering the eye, the melanin in the stromal melanocytes and also the melanin pigment in the epithelium. We know that melanin is important because in albino people, who do not have any melanin pigment, the iris is pink, the rich stromal blood supply providing the only colour.

A blue iris has an epithelium full of melanin but only a meagre dusting of melanin granules in the melanocytes. White light is a spectrum ranging from short wavelength, low-energy, blue light to long wavelength, higher-energy, red light. The longer wavelength red light has little trouble passing through the stroma but it is absorbed by the heavily pigmented epithelium. The short wavelength low-energy light, on the other hand, is scattered by the fine, particulate components which make up the iris stroma and so the iris is seen as being blue. Brown eyes have lots of melanin in their stromal melanocytes and also there is the front border region where the melanocytes are close together and full of melanin. The heavy-pigmented stroma is seen as brown. Hazel, green and grey eyes have progressively less stromal pigment than brown eyes and fit in between the two eye colour extremes. In brown irises, each melanocyte has more melanin than is found in green or blue irises but it is more controversial whether or not they have more melanocytes. In a newborn baby's iris, melanin production has not got into full swing so their eyes are blue or grey.

Aqueous humour

Aqueous humour is the clear fluid which provides the lens cells and the corneal endothelium with nutrition and also is responsible for keeping the eye inflated. It is produced continuously by structures called the *ciliary processes* which are located behind the iris and close by the lens (Plate 2). The origin of the fluid is blood plasma which leaks from fine blood vessels (called capillaries) at the centre of each process, but it is modified by secretory epithelial cells lining the process. This means that aqueous humour has similar constituents to blood plasma, although in different proportions. Vitamin C, for example, is around 20 times higher in the aqueous humour than in blood plasma, although as yet no one really knows why we need so much vitamin C inside the eye.

The aqueous humour passes between the lens and the iris, then through the pupil and enters the *anterior chamber* at the front of the eye lined by the cornea and the front surface of the iris (Plate 2). As aqueous humour is continuously formed at around 2–4 microlitres each minute, it must also continuously escape from the eye at the same rate. The turnover of aqueous humour is such that its whole volume is replaced about five to six times each day. The fluid gets back into blood vessels and out of the eye by modified structures located in the limbus where the clear cornea changes into the white sclera. The drain is known as the *outflow system* of the eye (Figure 1.6). The outflow system consists of a filter region called the *trabecular meshwork*, a single collecting vessel (*Schlemm's canal*) and a series of fine channels leading the clear aqueous humour back into the blood supply at the conjunctiva. The natural resistance offered by the drain restricts fluid passage and builds up the back pressure of around 16 mm of mercury necessary to keep the eye inflated and maintain its shape. Think of a dam on a river: flow of water through the dam is restricted and a lake develops – the lake of the eye is the anterior chamber filled with aqueous humour (Figure 1.3 and Plate 2). If the drain becomes partially blocked as happens in *glaucoma*, then eye pressure is elevated pathologically (see chapter 3).

Lens

The lens lies behind the pupil. Partly covered by the iris (Figure 1.3 and Plate 2), it is made up of a mass of elongated cells which form ever-tighter layers towards the centre. The construction is much like the layers of an onion, but unlike the spherical onion the lens has a far more elliptical (rugby ball) shape. Also unlike an onion, the lens grows from the outside inwards so that the oldest part of the lens is right at its centre. Over the cellular onion is a layer of material rather like the basement membranes mentioned earlier, only much thicker. The thick layer of material is called the *capsule*.

The lens is held in place by thin threads of robust material called *zonules* which attach the capsule to a structure known as the *ciliary body*. The ciliary processes which produce aqueous humour extend from this structure, and it also houses the *ciliary muscle*. The latter is a large and complicated smooth muscle which, through its contraction and relaxation, adjusts the tension in the zonules and hence alters the shape of the lens. Such fine tuning alterations are necessary for *accommodation* whereby both faraway and near-at-hand objects can be brought into focus on the retina.

THE BACK OF THE EYE

Vitreous humour

The large cavity at the back of the eye (Figure 1.3), making up four-fifths of its volume, is filled with a clear jelly-like substance called the *vitreous humour* which has the same consistency as egg white. The vitreous humour serves to protect the delicate retina by providing it with support and cushioning – nature's bubble wrap. Like all other structures in the optical pathway to the retina, it is transparent.

Retinal blood supply

When you look normally at the pupil of the eye, it is black. If a bright light is pointed at the eye, the pupil will narrow of course, but the back of the eye will now appear red. The *red reflex* is not showing up the retina, because that has to be transparent to let the light through to the vision receptors. What you are seeing is the red of the massive blood supply that feeds the busy retina: it has blood vessels on it, in it and a vast supply behind it in the *choroid* (Figure 1.3, Plates 4 and 13). The red reflex is of course the *red eye* which spoils the effect of many amateur flash photographs.

The blood in the choroid surges under the outer retina and is one of the fastest blood flows in the body. The retina needs a fast and efficient blood supply because of the high energy demands of vision, as regards both the need for nutrition and the elimination of waste products. In some animals, such as the guinea pig, the retina is sufficiently thin that all the nutritional requirements can be provided by the choroid. In primates, including humans, the retina is much thicker and so, on the vitreal side (conventionally the inner retina), it requires an additional supply which comes through the *optic nerve head.*

Retina

Histological sections through the retina show it to be a complex but orderly arrangement of nervous tissue which can be seen in Figure 1.7. The retina is an elaborate circuit board where light is converted into electrical signals prior to these signals being conducted to the brain to be turned into vision (see chapter 2). The specialized cells, or *photoreceptors,* which convert light into signals are called *rods* and *cones* (Figure 1.7). The names relate to their appearance, with rods being thin pencil-like structures whereas cones are much fatter (Figure 1.8). In humans, the receptors are situated in the retina at the furthest point away from the light. This is why the retina has to be clear, otherwise we would not see too well. Strangely, this suboptimal

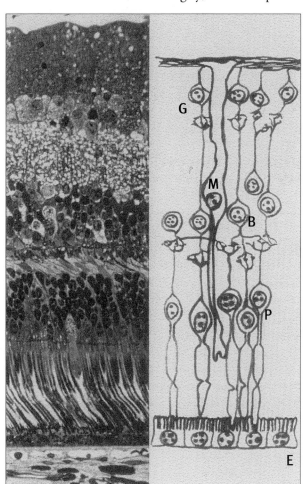

Figure 1.7 Stained section through the retina with a drawing of the connecting nerves. Ganglion cell layer (G), Müller cell (M), bipolar cells (B), rod and cone photoreceptors (P) and retinal pigment epithelium (E) can be seen. (*Provided by Dr Luminita Paraoan, University of Liverpool*)

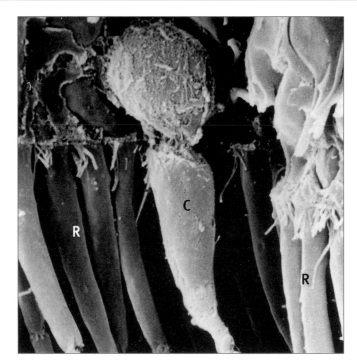

Figure 1.8   Rods (R) and cones (C) as seen under the electron
microscope. An eye built on this scale would fill a football pitch!

arrangement is present in all animals with backbones. Some other animals, such as squid and octopus, have their photoreceptors at the front of the 'circuit board' and, although their eyes are quite different from our own, they benefit from vision that is truly superb.

In our own system, cones are the photoreceptors which work in the light; they are concerned with colour and sharpness of vision. Rods give black-and-white vision without fine detail, but they do not need as much light as the cones to be effective (for more detail see chapter 2). The human retina has far fewer cones than rods and they are not evenly distributed. Indeed there is a 5 mm in diameter circular spot on the retina which contains an unusually high density of cones. At the very centre of this spot, the *macula* (see Plate 4), is a pit or depression, termed the *fovea*, where the retina is very thin (Figure 1.9). Here there is very little other than cones. The lens focuses light on the macula and it is this region which is responsible for our high visual acuity and so-called central vision.

The rod, the receptor of most use in darkness, consists of a main cell body from which extends the *outer segment*, a thin cylinder filled with membranous discs (Figure 1.10). The cylinder and discs are in structure very like the stacks of coins wrapped in paper that you may sometimes see

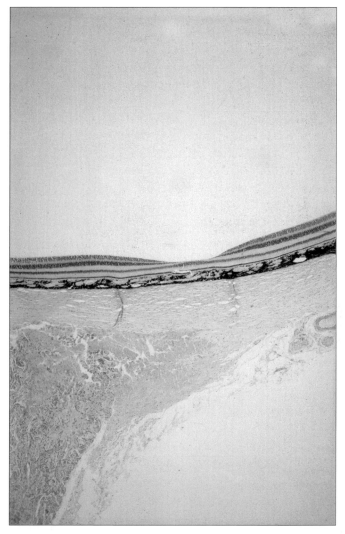

Figure 1.9 A stained section through the retina in the region of the
macula. The pit formed by the fovea can be seen.

in a bank or a till. The disc membranes of the outer segment are where
all the action takes place – it is here that light bleaches visual pigment,
thus initiating the first event in the electrochemical process which culminates
in vision. The visual pigment of the rod is called *rhodopsin* and a key player
in the process of bleaching is a derivative of vitamin A present in the visual
pigment. The derivative is related to beta-carotene found in carrots and
through this relationship came the tale that 'carrots help you see in the
dark'.

The cone has a much plumper and prominent outer segment (Figure 1.8) which contains a mass of membranes, but not in the form of the discrete discs seen in the rod. Instead the membrane is continuous but still serves as a template where photobleaching takes place. The visual pigments on the membranes within the outer segments of cones are different from rhodopsin but they require the same derivative of vitamin A. Also, like the rhodopsin of rods, the visual pigments of cones are bleached by light. However, there are separate populations of cones with pigments that have different sensitivities within the light spectrum, and so we can identify red, green and blue – the basis of colour discrimination.

The photoreceptors, both rods and cones, connect on their inner aspect with a layer of nerve cells of various types, the main one being a *bipolar cell*. In turn the bipolar cells and their associates link up with a second set of retinal nerves called the *ganglion cells*, and so the electrochemical messages pass through the retina from one cell type to another (Figure 1.7). Ganglion cells have nerve fibres which extend over the surface of the retina and meet at the optic nerve head (see later). Holding the whole elegantly structured tissue together are *Müller cells*, which are a type of *glia* (support cells in brain tissue). A second type of glia, the *astrocyte*, is closely associated with the small blood vessels which feed the inner retina.

Retinal pigment epithelium

We moved from the photoreceptors of the outer retina to the ganglion cells of the inner retina in the last section. If, from the photoreceptors, we move the other way towards the choroid, we meet at the base of the outer segments a single layer of cells which make up the *retinal pigment epithelium* (Figures 1.7 and 1.10). These epithelial cells rest on a complex matrix layer called *Bruch's membrane* separating them from the blood vessels of the choroid. The pigment epithelium is an unusual cell which has many functions, all of which are vital to vision.

This epithelium is the nursemaid of the rods and cones, and its main role is to keep the photoreceptors and the visual process in tip-top condition. It is important to note that the rods and cones do not undergo cellular division, so they are never replaced: those you have when you are young are all you will ever have. Rods and cones have to last a lifetime, unlike other parts of the body, for example skin, which has a turnover time of between two and four weeks, or the lining epithelium of the gut, which is replaced every three to five days. As they are so precious, the photoreceptors need to be cared for and it is the retinal pigment epithelium that does all the pampering.

As the rod's outer segment discs become worn out by the continuous activity, new ones are produced by the *inner segment* of the main cell body.

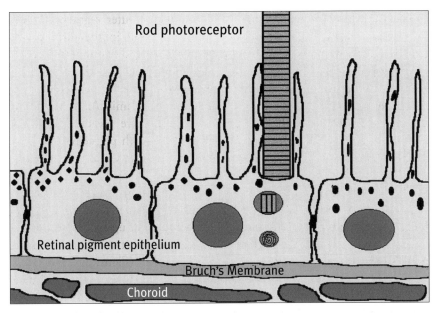

Figure 1.10 A diagram of the retinal pigment epithelium. This nursemaid cell eats bits off the rods (and cones) to keep them in tip-top condition.

The further away the disc is from the main photoreceptor body, the older it is, so those that snuggle up to the retinal pigment epithelial cells are the oldest (Figure 1.10). The outer segments do not become bigger and bigger, simply because the pigment epithelium nips off the oldest ones in the stack (in the rods) or ribbon (in the cones). I like to compare the stack of discs in the rod outer segment to those very symmetrical crisps that come in a cardboard tube. All the epithelial cell does is to take the bottom few crisps (discs) in the stack and 'eat' them. The discs taken inside the cell are digested with enzymes (digestive juices) and the remnants are extruded, initially into Bruch's membrane and thereafter passing into the choroidal circulation (Figure 1.10).

It may seem perverse that a cell which is supposed to look after the photoreceptors is forever eating them, but there is another way of looking at the process. Your photoreceptors are the same age as you are, but the oldest disc is only 14 days old. This is the time it takes for an epithelial cell to eat its way through the whole stack of discs, and of course by then the whole lot have been renewed.

The epithelial cells do not snack, but have one 'main meal' per day, first thing in the morning. When you wake up and put the light on or open the curtains, it is then that the epithelium sets about biting off the spent discs from the stack. After another day of vision, the epithelium is ready the next morning to take another bite. How the epithelial cells co-ordinate their eating habits so precisely is still unknown, but a daily rhythm of this kind is called a *circadian rhythm* and examples from elsewhere in the body include such things as blood pressure level and breathing rate.

I have for the most part been describing the relationship between the rod and the epithelium. The same process takes place with cones, but retinal pigment epithelial cells eat the end of a continuous strip rather than the package of discrete discs associated with the rod. Also the process is slower and is more active at night rather than in the morning. If rod photoreceptor discs are imagined as crisps, the cone material can be seen as folded lasagna, but no matter what we compare outer segment material to, the epithelium certainly eats its fill. It is unknown how much cone material is eaten in a lifetime, but each epithelial cell consumes in excess of 100 million rod discs.

The retinal pigment epithelium also performs other functions. It is pigmented and, with the choroid, it is part of the blackout curtain which prevents stray light from reflecting back into the receptor system. The cells also store vitamin A for the visual process and they supply dietary essentials to the photoreceptors. An important function is to act as a dam to prevent blood and plasma from the leaky choroidal vessels penetrating into the retina. The cells are not a complete barrier because they selectively allow some plasma constituents access while holding back others. All in all, the epithelial cells control the environment in which the rods and cones live and act as their servants throughout the photoreceptors', hopefully, long lives.

Optic nerve

Using a light, the eye doctor or optician looking into the interior of the eye through the pupil sees the red reflex, and with some magnification (perhaps from an ophthalmoscope; see chapter 3) can identify, by looking centrally, a white circle in the sea of red. More magnification will show blood vessels extending from the white circle like red branches from a tree, and perhaps the macula will be visible as a spot close by (Plate 4). The white area is the optic nerve head which is the start point of the nerve that links the eye and the brain.

The electrical message generated from light by the rods and cones which passes through the retina to the ganglion cells then travels along the optic nerve to reach the brain. In fact the optic nerve is the conduit for long thin threads called nerve fibres which track from the ganglion cells spread all over the retina to meet up and form bundles in the optic nerve head. A little over one million of these fibres come together at the nerve head to extend in an orderly manner down the nerve. If you think of spaghetti in a pasta jar, the nerve bundles are the spaghetti and the nerve is the jar.

The optic nerve extends from the eye, across the orbit, through an opening at the base of the orbit and meets up with the nerve from the other eye at the *chiasma*. The nerves then separate again and track to the *visual cortex* on the right and left sides of the brain. The visual cortex and what it does will be covered in the next chapter.

FACTS AND OLD WIVES' TALES

✧ Blinking takes place without us thinking about it, but if we try to stop blinking we can do it for a minute or so but not much more. Not all animals need to blink; for example, rabbits blink rarely if at all.

✧ The human retina has nearly 20 times as many rods as cones; there are about 125 million rods and fewer than 7 million cones.

✧ 'Your eyes are as blue as the sky and as deep as the ocean' may only be a feeble chat-up line but it sounds better than the factual 'Your eyes are blue because the iris scatters short wavelength light, just like the sky and the sea.'

✧ 'Carrots help you see in the dark.' It is true that carrots contain beta-carotene, which is closely related to one of the essential compounds that make rods function, and rods are the photoreceptors that function most efficiently in dim light. For most of us the beta-carotene from carrots, tomatoes or other vegetables makes no difference to our night vision, which is as good as it can be. However, for those people who are night blind due to deficiency in vitamin A, a boost of beta-carotene from carrots can make a difference to what they see in dim light.

Chapter 2

Eye see!
The mechanism of vision

Sight is a double act performed by the eye and the brain, with the eye converting light into modified electrochemical impulses while the brain converts those impulses into pictures. The double act is extremely complicated and far from understood, but in this chapter I will try to deal with the main principles of the amazing mechanism of vision.

VISION AT THE RETINA

Human beings have two different seeing skills: the dominant one is *central vision*, but there is another called *side* (or peripheral) *vision*. As explained in the previous chapter, we also have two different classes of photoreceptors, the rods and cones. In this section we will find out a little more about sight and the retina.

Central versus side vision

Central vision is the dominant form of vision in humans and it is concentrated around the macula, the spot in the retina where there is a high concentration of cones (see Plate 4). As the receptor involved in colour vision and seeing things sharply, the cone needs a lot of light in order to work properly. Thus central vision is daylight vision, and the light-focusing tissues of the eye (the cornea and lens) make sure the central region and the macular region in particular have more than their fair share of the light that is available.

Side vision is the province of most of the retina, in fact all the retina outside a narrow ring around the macula. Although there are some cones, this part of the retina is the domain of the rod. The rod cannot recognize colour and rod-dominated vision is associated with rather fuzzy images, but the rod has the great advantage of being able to work in low levels of light. Side vision is the vision of the night, or rather twilight for humans, because we do need some light in order to see.

To demonstrate the difference between central and side vision, take two coins and look at them on a table in front of you in reasonable lighting conditions. Shut one eye and concentrate with the other on the two coins. This is pure central vision in operation. Lower your head if you need to, to see all the fine detail on the coins. Now start moving the right-hand coin to the right, just a little, and then stop; then a little more and then stop, and so on. Keep concentrating on the left-hand coin to see the fine detail. It is hard to resist tracking along with the right-hand coin (*central dominance* in action), but you can do it. You don't have to move the right-hand coin very far to see the fine detail on it go fuzzy, so now you are seeing the left coin with central vision and the right coin with side vision (seeing out of the corner of your eye). There is a huge difference in the quality of the image. On the other hand, you really have to move the coin quite a distance for it to go out of range altogether. So, central vision dominates but has an extremely narrow effective field, whereas side vision is passive but has a very large field of operation. This field is the *visual field*, which widens the further the object is from the eye.

It is an important point that we are not born with good central vision and central dominance; these develop after birth and need proper light stimulation. If the macula is not stimulated by sufficient light, central visual development can slow down or stop altogether. If, as happens on rare occasions, a child is born with a dense cataract so that the lens is completely opaque (see chapter 4), then until the cataractous lens is removed, proper visual development is at risk. Also in children with certain types of squint central vision can be endangered in the squinting eye (see chapters 3 and 4).

Photopic (day) and scotopic (night) vision

The two types of receptor work best in different lighting conditions. In bright light cones do all the work (*photopic vision*) and in very dim conditions only a rod can work (*scotopic vision*). This does not mean that the two systems never work together – there is a broad range of lighting conditions where this occurs (*mesopic vision*). In the midday sun, vision is by cones, while only rods can cope with a dark night, but in full moonlight or at dusk you are in the mesopic range where some colour can still be made out.

If you enter a darkened room after being in the bright light, you can see nothing. Only after a while will you start to see detail and it can take up to 30 minutes to become fully dark-adapted. This is how long it takes for all the rods to kick into top gear. Think about what it is like when you first go into a cinema. The usher takes your ticket, shines a torch on to it and strides off or points confidently towards your seat. You on the other hand can see very little and may stumble over people's feet or spray popcorn over everyone. Eventually you get settled down and slowly your pupils dilate, letting in as much of the available dim light as possible to the retina; as your rods start to reach threshold you can make out the frowning faces round about and wonder why you couldn't see this well just a few moments ago. Rods are just no good at detail, making the scotopic world one of movement and blurry shapes, so it is just as well that the photopic system of cones kicks back in when you look at the bright screen to enjoy the film. Central dominance takes over as you concentrate on the action scene, but you may become vaguely aware of movement at the edge of your visual field: someone else has just come into the cinema and it is their turn to stumble around all over the place.

People can have great difficulties coping with dim lighting and the dark, and this, for some, is due to illnesses which affect either their side vision (as in glaucoma, for example) or their rods (as in some forms of *retinitis pigmentosa*) (see chapter 4). Vitamin A deficiency can result in *night blindness* because of the lack of the modified form of vitamin A that joins with a protein to form the visual pigment required for the rods to function. However, some people are born night blind; these people exhibit a defect in the transmission of electrochemical signals from the photoreceptors to the other retinal cells. Both receptor systems are defective, but the rods are worse than the cones.

Colour vision

I have mentioned colour vision already, but now let us take the opportunity to examine how it might work. All sorts of people have tried to study and understand how we see colour, including physiologists, anatomists, physicists, neurologists, psychologists, physicians, metaphysicians and scholars of many persuasions, and this has led to there being many speculations but little concrete proof. Therefore much of this section is based on the favourite theory of the present time, the *trichromatic theory*, which is a working model of how colour vision might work but still remains speculative.

This trichrome (three colours) proposal suggests that the retina contains three types of cone which respond differently to the available light. White light is made up of light of different wavelengths mixed together, which separates out in, for example, a rainbow, with blue light being of short wavelength and red at the other extreme being of long. In effect the retina is said to have blue cones, green cones and red cones; the blue respond best to short wavelengths, green to the middle of the range and red to the long wavelengths. All other colours are explained by appropriate mixes of the cone types working in conjunction in much the same way as an artist would mix paints on a palette to create the correct colour.

In general, *colour blindness* should more accurately be known as *colour defectiveness* and it is far more common in people of European descent than it is in either Asians or Africans. It is preponderantly males who are colour defective with around 8 per cent of males and only 0.5 per cent of females in Europe experiencing colour discrimination problems. Colour defects occur when one or more of the cone types do not function or function poorly. The loss of function or the inadequate functioning is a consequence of an absence or lack of the photopigment in the appropriate cone type(s). As a result colour defectiveness ranges from having minor difficulties in distinguishing some shades of red from some shades of green to a profound inability to distinguish colour of any sort. This extreme situation is fortunately rare but having some form of minor defect is common.

If you have a minor defect, you are 'colour anomalous', and it is more than probable you don't even know about it as the defect will be so subtle that it is unlikely to have any influence on your life other than as a result of curiosity value. I am particularly conscious of this because, although I have worked and taught in hospital and university eye departments all my adult life, I was completely unaware that I have a red/green anomaly until I started researching this book. It was not until I was checked out on a very sensitive colour vision machine called an *anomaloscope* that I was found not to have perfect colour vision. I can see red and I can see green, but I can't distinguish some reddish/greens from greenish/reds.

Colour defectiveness, on the other hand, is more profound and can be a handicap in some professions, for example those related to art and design, and is even a safety problem for aircraft pilots and some jobs in the navy. Colour defectiveness is a bar to working as a railway driver or linesman. The types of colour defect are as follows:

✧ protanopia (first) – a red colour problem;

✧ deuteranopia (second) – a green colour problem; and

✧ tritanopia (third) – a blue colour problem.

Defects in red and green vision are considerably more common than a blue colour problem, which tends to be a rarity.

Red/green colour defectiveness is an inherited condition carried on the X-chromosome which determines gender, so the defect is described as being sex-linked. Also the particular genes involved in colour vision on the X-chromosome are recessive, which means that the colour defect will not come into effect in a female (she has two X-chromosomes – XX) unless both carry the defect. A male, on the other hand, is XY and has only one X-chromosome, so if this X-chromosome carries the defect then it will be expressed. So for a woman both parents would have to carry the defect for her to have a colour vision problem, whereas a man needs only his mother (who gives him his X-chromosome) to be a carrier. In this way you would expect far more men to exhibit colour defects and anomalies than women, as is the case.

Colour vision testing is not complicated and the most common way is to use an *Ishihara chart* (Plate 5). The chart comprises coloured dots of equal brightness, and in consistent lighting conditions individuals either succeed (normal) or fail (colour defective or anomalous) to recognize a particular number made up of coloured dots against a different coloured background. There are other variations on this theme, but a different style of test altogether is the *Lantern test*, in which a series of appropriate coloured lights are shown in succession that then have to be accurately identified. This test is particularly relevant for aircraft pilots and is often required in industries where reliable identification of lights has safety implications. The anomaloscope mentioned earlier is a rather expensive machine not really used in common practice, being more a research instrument for identifying minor anomalies.

Visual acuity

The dual characteristics of the photopic system are colour vision and good *visual acuity*. Visual acuity is technically the resolving power of the eye to make out form, i.e. discrimination. Good acuity means that a shape, will be crisp or sharp, while poor acuity makes the shape's outline blurred. One reason why the cone is better than the rod at discriminating is that in the central region there is almost one ganglion cell for each cone whereas in the marginal region (providing side vision) there are many hundreds of rods to each ganglion cell. As the nerve fibres of ganglion cells are responsible for the transmission of the electrochemical messages to the brain, the relatively poor service available to the rods compared with the cones must be significant.

In practice, visual acuity is judged by the ability of central vision to discriminate objects as being separate or alternatively to identify familiar forms. Obviously we are better at doing this with close objects than those far away, so distance counts. At distances shorter than 6 metres (20 feet) accommodation comes into play, so the 'gold standard' test of visual acuity, the *Snellen chart*, is set at that distance. This chart is commonly seen in the doctor's office or optician's shop and consists of a white chart lit from the front or box lit from within which has black letters; the larger letters are at the top, becoming smaller and more numerous as you go down the list (Figure 2.1).

One eye is tested at a time with the other eye covered. The largest letter should be distinguished by someone with good vision at 60 metres; the smallest, which stretches even the best vision at 6 metres, is sized for reading at 4 metres. If you can read the second line from the bottom, it indicates

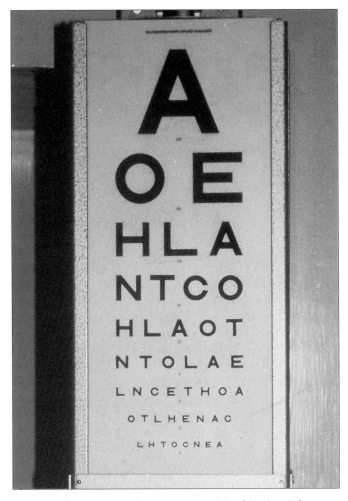

Figure 2.1 The Snellen chart to test vision (visual acuity).

that you have 6/6 vision, or in the USA, where they measure in feet rather than metres, 20/20 vision; both mean the same thing – your visual acuity is excellent. All the test does is establish what good discrimination should be at a given distance and test how close you come to it.

Another way of doing the same thing would be to have letters all of the same size, move you to a point where the letters were fuzzy and then bring you in closer until you could see them. A person with good visual acuity would end up further away from the screen than someone with poor acuity.

The 6/12 line equates roughly with what is needed for the UK driving test, reading a car numberplate at 25 yards (22.9 metres), while seeing solely the top letter on the Snellen chart from 6 metres gives only 6/60 vision, which would be a marked visual limitation. Further stages for those with visual weakness are to test the top letter at 3 metres (3/60), then the doctor would come in to one metre away and ask the subject to count the number of fingers held up (count fingers, CF), to detect the movement of a waving hand (hand movements, HM) and finally, if vision is minimal, to perceive light (PL). For blind registration, the best seeing eye is 3/60 or worse with glasses correction. Although the Snellen test usually involves looking at letters, my eye doctor and optometrist colleagues remind me that what is being tested is not reading, so your reading glasses are not required. The test can also be with different sizes of the letter E; the subject has to say which way the letter is facing. Very similar is the *Landolt C test*, which involves different sizes of this letter in different positions and the subject is required to say where the break in the C is located.

Astigmatism

Astigmatism is a visual failing brought about usually because of imperfections in the curve of the corneal surface which make the bending of light (refraction) uneven in different parts of the cornea. You can be born with some astigmatism or you can develop it because of corneal problems such as injury or scarring. Surgery to the eye, for example corneal grafting, cataract and glaucoma operations, can produce unwanted astigmatism. Another cause of astigmatism is if the lens within the eye, the natural one or the plastic form introduced at cataract surgery, is not quite in the ideal position. Appropriate correction for astigmatism is incorporated into your glasses or contact lenses by the optometrist (see chapter 3).

FOCUSING LIGHT

In chapter 1, I introduced you to the tissues concerned with focusing light on the retina (the cornea and lens) and also those controlling the amount of light entering the inner reaches of the eye (iris and pupil). In this section, we will deal with refraction and accommodation, which are the stock in trade of the structures at the front of the eye, and binocular vision, which is the result of a combination of tissues including those at the front of the eye.

Refraction

Refraction basically is the bending of light rays when light passes through one clear material to another, such as happens between air and glass or air and water. For example, if you are looking into a rockpool at the seaside and quickly reach down into it for a shell or a pebble, usually you will miss because your eyes are being fooled and the object is not quite where you think it is. If you try a second time, but more slowly, the part of your

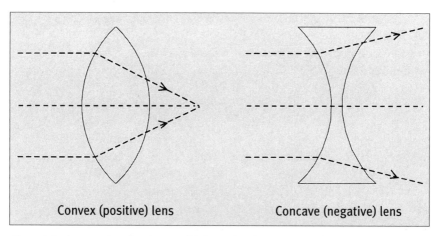

Figure 2.2 A convex lens bends rays of light so that they come together, whereas a concave lens bends them away.

arm under water seems as if it is bent a little to one side, but now it is much easier to locate the object you are after. Light rays are bent between air and water by refraction and so the image of the shell or pebble is displaced slightly to one side.

If, on the other hand, light rays pass into and then through a curved object, then its shape will also contribute to the bending of the light. A bowed out or convex structure will tend to bend light rays so that they come together, and a bevelled in or concave structure does the opposite (Figure 2.2; see also Figure 3.5); glass and plastic lenses are of both types. The bending of light is measured in *dioptres* (D), with a plus figure (+1D, etc.) being a measure of how much light rays are being bent to converge together and a minus figure (–1D, etc.) being a measure of how much they are bent to spread away from each other. (More will be said on this subject in the section on glasses and contact lenses in chapter 3.)

The biological refractive systems of the eye are the cornea and the lens, and together they focus the parallel rays of light on the back of the eye. The clear cornea has a light-bending power of +43D, whereas the crystalline lens within the eye can range from +15D to +23D, so the cornea is by far the more important for bringing light rays together at the back of the eye. On the other hand, because the lens can change shape it is crucial for fine focus and accommodation.

Accommodation

Just bending light (refraction) is not good enough to obtain a clear retinal image, especially if near objects and those at a distance are to be seen equally well. For this it is necessary to have at least one refractive system which is

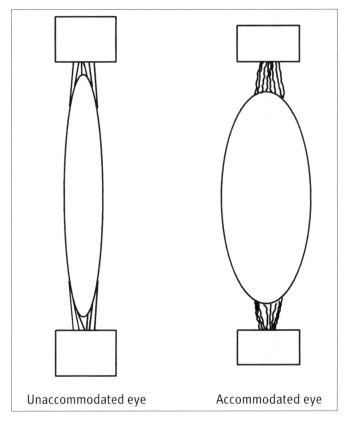

Unaccommodated eye   Accommodated eye

Figure 2.3 In the unaccommodated lens, the zonule threads which hold
the lens in place are taut and the lens is stretched and thin
(exaggerated here). During accommodation, the zonules become slack
and the lens becomes more spherical (a convex lens becoming more
positive) and thus can bend light more.

variable and that is the crystalline lens. The lens can vary its light-bending power by changing shape from being more spherical to being more oval and back again when needed.

The natural shape of the crystalline lens is relatively spherical and this is when its bending power is at its greatest, which is needed for near vision (about +23D ideally). The bending power is high because this is when the curve on the lens is greatest. You may remember from chapter 1 that the lens is suspended in the eye by a number of tough threads called zonules. The zonules stretch from the lens to the ciliary body which, as well as producing the aqueous humour, also houses a large muscle called the ciliary muscle.

The muscle fibres are arranged in such a way that when they contract they narrow the space between themselves and the lens so that the zonules are not under tension. In this circumstance the lens is not under tension either, so the elastic cover around the lens, called the capsule (see chapter 1), is free to alter the lens into the more rounded or spherical shape ideal for near vision. Relaxation of the ciliary muscle is required for distance vision. As the muscle relaxes, it moves further away from the lens and the zonules start to stretch and flatten out the pliable lens. This decreases its curvature and also its refractive power, the latter down to the minimum of +15D which is needed for a sharp image at distance (Figure 2.3).

Binocular vision

The eyes in humans and many other primates are at the front of the head and not at the side as, for example, in sheep, zebra and deer. As mentioned in chapter 1, having eyes at the side of the head gives an extremely wide field of vision, but humans sacrifice this for another advantage, and have to put up with the bother of turning their heads to see behind. The advantage of having two eyes pointing ahead is that their respective visual fields overlap, and where they overlap we get binocularity.

The brain receives two slightly different images of any object that both right and left eyes are looking at and these are fused to make one image.

A good three-dimensional (3D) or stereo image is of huge practical advantage to humans, apes and monkeys because it gives good *depth perception.* Primates in general need a good sense of depth and without the ability to place objects in a three-dimensional pattern many activities would be far more difficult. An obvious advantage of good stereo vision is the ability of monkeys and apes to swing through the branches of trees; we marvel at the gibbon's aerial agility, none of which would be practical without binocular vision. Good hand-to-eye co-ordination supported by a fused stereo image gives us huge practical advantages. For example, threading a needle is a difficult enough task with two eyes (stereo) and a totally impractical proposition with one eye closed (mono).

A bang on the head or too much alcohol can give rise to temporary *double vision* because fusion of the image is not taking place. A more permanent double vision can occur in patients with squint (see chapter 4). The fusion process takes place in the brain and, although not everything we see with our two eyes is fused, the brain also has the fortunate ability to suppress double images that would otherwise confuse so that we are not aware of them. These double images are easy to show if we trick the eye and brain. Look at a picture on the wall or something in the distance. Bring up a finger about a foot away from your nose and it will look like two. Now stare at the finger rather than the picture, and the finger will be one and the picture two.

Looking with one eye only does not give an impression of a flat two-dimensional (2D) world, because we still get depth perception with one eye, although it is not as good as with two. This is achieved through a variety of clues which tell us about 'near things' and 'far things'. An example is that colour gives us a sense of distance – distant mountains appear blue due to scattering of light by the atmosphere, so if something is blue and hazy then we perceive it as being far away (see also the next section on eye and brain). Haziness or blurring is an important distance clue. How many times have you heard someone say that something in the distance looks closer than normal? I enjoy looking from Birkenhead across the River Mersey to the main landmarks of Liverpool, the Liver Building and the two cathedrals. On a hazy or bleak day they are away in the distance, but some days, days when the atmosphere is clear and the buildings are sharper to the eye, I swear I could just reach out and touch them.

There are many other clues that help with distance, whether seen with one or two eyes, such as the size of familiar objects. If a cottage is small, it is in the distance, and if it is big, it is close by. We know that the smaller fence posts are in the distance and the larger are nearer. The artist creates the illusion of 3D on a 2D canvas by introducing perspective, the trick of painting things in the distance smaller than those that are meant to be close by. The church art of the early Middle Ages looks strange because the artists did not use perspective in their works and therefore they did not achieve the distinctions between 'near' and 'far' that we take for granted. Shadows are also very important in giving an object a solid appearance.

Artists also create 3D effects by introducing light and dark areas on to their objects to represent light and shade. This works because light and shade are powerful clues about shape, depth and 3D structure to us. Look at the two circles in Figure 2.4. One is an ordinary circle with even shading and the other circle has speckles in it; because the speckles are crude shading, the second circle has depth and can be seen as a ball even if it is examined with one eye closed. A form of camouflage used by four-legged animals is to have a light belly and a dark back as protective shading. During the day, shade will make the belly look darker and direct sun will lighten the back. Protective shading makes an animal look uniformly coloured at a distance so helping it to appear flat and blend into the background. Colouring to look flat is not just a feature of exotic animals such as tigers and wildebeest, but can be seen nearer to home on foxes, some cattle and donkeys.

EYE AND BRAIN

The relationship between the eye and the brain is a huge subject area which goes well beyond the scope of this book. It has been written about at length in popular science books and I would recommend either *Eye and Brain* by

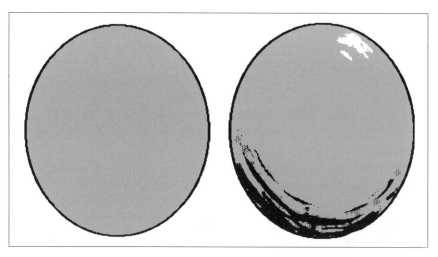

Figure 2.4 The circle on the left has uniform colouring, but if shading at the bottom and highlighting at the top are introduced, the circle starts to look like a ball (3D effect).

R. Gregory or S.M. Zeki's *A Vision of the Brain* for those who have more than a passing interest (see Further Reading at the end of the book for full references). It may be fair to say, in summary, that painstaking and detailed research confirms the complexity and flexibility of the system. Much remains a mystery about the relationship between the retina and the brain and particularly about the visual process. Here I will mention only a few aspects, dipping into a field too vast to be represented properly by the casual approach of this book.

Visual cortex

The visual cortex is that part of the brain where visual signals generated in the retina are processed. The visual cortex is responsible for visual perception but it is not the only part of the brain involved in the visual process in its broadest sense. A number of other areas have been identified, each having distinctive functions or functions in common with other areas that relate to the visual experience, such as spatial perception, discrimination and recognition.

The cortex is particularly important in human beings for without it there is complete blindness; the eye's only response to light in this circumstance is narrowing of pupil diameter. This is not the case for all animals. Monkeys without the visual cortex have profound visual defects but are not blind, while rabbits have some visual impairment but they still can avoid obstacles placed in their path. Removal of the visual cortex from reptiles and birds hardly diminishes their visual capabilities. In evolution towards primates the cortex became progressively more important for vision, until in humans it was the exclusive organ for visual perception and the main visual reactions such as accommodation, fusion of the two images and fixation.

Visual perception

An important part of how humans function visually is the strange business of *visual perception*, which is the brain processing ocular and other sensory information and making a 'best guess' with regard to what the eyes are looking at. Visual perception has an elusive characteristic in that, as Professor R. L. Gregory put it, 'it goes beyond the available sensory evidence'.

When you look with central vision at an object close at hand in good lighting conditions you can be aware of every detail, but this is not always the case. More often than not something is recognized in less than ideal circumstances with a minimum of visual evidence. 'Who is that in the distance?' 'What is that at the back of the dark cupboard?' 'Which animal ran past at great speed?' It becomes apparent that we need a mechanism to cope with minimal or confusing visual input – well-being and, at times, survival may depend on it. 'That is an enemy in the distance!' 'I think I see a mouse trap at the back of the cupboard!' 'There are mountain lions around here!'

Patterns of perception require taking the visual information from the cortex and integrating it with other sensations. Of particular importance is visual memory and then making a best 'photofit' against a 'photograph album' locked away in the visual memory bank. The visual information may be insufficient initially, but after staring hard and seeing more of the subject a match can be made. Imagine for a moment two people having a conversation about a third person way off in the distance.

> 'Who is that way over there, creeping up on us?' ['Who' not 'what', because its shape is perceived as human, already the process has begun.]
>
>   'It's a young lad. Do we know him?' [More visual detail is available about clothes, height, etc.]
>
>   'No, it's not young Gary from High Farm! You must be blind!' [A disagreement on photofit.] 'Ah, it's our Terry, I'd know him any-where!' [More information on facial detail, hair colouring, build and then a better photofit.]

Looking at drawings and paintings requires the perceptual process for interpretation. A few lines on a page are a few lines on a page, but drawn in a certain pattern they are perceived as a box. An outer circle with some strategically drawn inner circles and ovals becomes a face (Plate 6). Think of warm summer days, looking at clouds and seeing castles and dragons, or on cold winter nights recognizing beautiful pictures in the living-room fire. Seeing pictures in clouds and through flames in a fire are the desperate

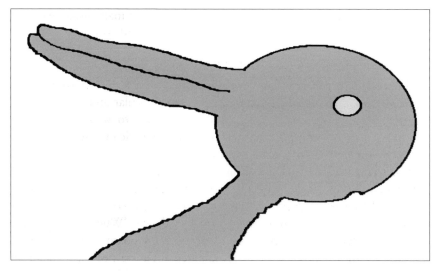

Figure 2.5 Looking one way the figure is a rabbit with long ears; looking the other way the ears become the bill of a duck.

attempts of the brain to identify something within its photograph album that would fit with such hazy images.

Ambiguous figures like the well-known Rubin's vase provide insufficient information for a clear photofit so the brain tries two different matches: sometimes you see two faces nose-to-nose and at other times you see a vase. I have used here another illustration, the less well-known ambiguous figure which looks like either a rabbit or a duck (Figure 2.5). Perception also comes into practised reading: you do not spell out each word as you read; rather the brain learns the shape of the words, giving you reading speed but often at the expense of missing obvious spelling mistakes. People do this all the time, reading and re-reading documents and missing obvious spelling errors because their minds see the words they expect to be there, not what really is there.

VISION IN ANIMALS

Light irritation and the directional response to light are basic properties of living things. Plants and plant cells have a light response, but it is in animals that specific organs have developed. The simplest organs merely located light and served as direction finders. Jellyfish, which are complex colonies of specialized cells, position themselves in the sea where their food is: too deep and they miss their prey, but too close to the surface and they will be buffeted by every wave. They solve their depth problem in part by using light cues, but this isn't strictly vision.

As animals became more biologically complex through evolution, there was a need for far more complex direction finders or senses. One type of direction finder became the eye. Different groups of animals solved the problem of sight in different ways and the mammalian eye is only one type of ocular sense organ. There are many blueprints for vision and even more variations on a given blueprint: cats' eyes and human eyes are variations on the theme of the mammalian ocular blueprint, such that the cat can see well at night and humans poorly, although this is reversed during daylight hours. In this section I will cover some features and curiosities from the different blueprints that nature has evolved for the many different groups of animals.

Primates and mammals

As the variations in lighting conditions over 24 hours are extreme, mammals, as with other groups of animals, have had to make compromises with the types of eyes they have developed, and these compromises relate to lifestyle. Humans have a daylight eye, and an exceptionally good daylight eye at that (photopic vision with cones; see earlier). It is not just a daylight eye, however, because we have rods (scotopic vision) to kick in for twilight vision, so extending the period of the day when we don't need aids like street lighting to see where we are going. Human rod-based vision is not particularly good and many animals have far better. Indeed for much of history, human beings were completely helpless at night beyond the range of a fire or a candle. We have only become a 24-hour species because first gas lamps and now electric lighting have created an artificial daytime for us.

A true night-time species is the cat, which has extremely well-developed night vision and can pick up minute movements with great accuracy in what to humans would be pitch darkness. Cats have a special structure called a tapetum at the back of the retina which reflects any light that passes through the retina back into it for use by the visual system: a 'waste-not want-not' principle. That is why cats' eyes glow in the dark when a torch beam is on them. Human eyes don't glow because they have a pigmented 'blackout screen' behind the retina to absorb stray light. This blackout screen is wasteful at night when it works against us, but comes into its own during daylight hours when it helps to achieve the clearest possible image.

The cat is in its visual element at night but during the day it has problems. The pupil must be closed down to a minimum because, with plenty of light available, the reflector works against good vision. The cat is easily dazzled. With a rod-based visual system and relatively few cones, cats cannot discriminate the fine detail that humans find easy; they are far less able to keep moving objects in sharp focus and the many colours and hues of our visual world are lost to them. Animals such as dogs, deer, cattle and so forth have tried to keep both options open, and as a consequence are nowhere near as good as the cat at night and do not come close to humans and monkeys for high-quality vision during the day. The cones they have give them a sense of form with regard to objects rather than colour vision as we know it.

Mammals with good or reasonably good night vision all need to close down their pupils as narrow as possible during the day. Technically it is more effective to close an oval pupil down to a slit in bright light than it is to close a circle down to a pinpoint. As a result a number of night-sighted animals such as goats, cats and dormice have developed oval pupils (Plate 7); the camel also gains considerable advantage from an oval pupil that reduces to a slit in the desert glare. Another group of animals, the seals, have oval pupils for an entirely different reason. Their eyes are adapted for seeing under water and have terrible astigmatism out of the water. The visual properties of their eyes are so bad that the only way they can see at all is to narrow the pupil down to a slit. As slit vision is necessary on land irrespective of lighting conditions, seals are one of the few groups of animals with voluntary control over their own pupil size.

Birds

The visual capabilities of birds can be truly amazing. The swallow at 3 miles up in the sky can see 60 miles in any direction. This is an important survival skill for a bird that has to cross the barren Sahara Desert during its 6,000-mile migration. The swallow needs to be able to pick out the infrequent green spots which are oases in the vast stretch of desert. If it misses a key watering hole, its body reserve of fluid may be insufficient to get it through. Even with such keen eyesight many of these little birds perish on their hazardous journey.

It is the birds of prey which are the true masters of vision. Birds in general are distinguished by having very thick well-organized retinas, but the retinas of birds of prey are even more pronounced. The hawk has over one million cones per square millimetre in the macula, which is five times that of the human. The large retinal network, plus the dense packing of cones, combine to give an awesome daylight visual response. The central visual acuity in hawks, buzzards and eagles is about eight times better than in humans. These birds make my claims about the power of the human eye seem rather feeble, but they need all their visual capabilities to pick out a small animal moving in the grass from where they hover high in the sky above.

One bird of prey with a different lifestyle is the nocturnal owl. They have big eyes with a very large lens and all sorts of adaptation to night hunting. Owls are generally considered to be colour blind, but some species are reputed to be able to see in the infra-red and even to be able to lock on to body heat rather like the high-tech night glasses that can see in pitch blackness. The owl is a flying 'night sight', but during the day most of them find a roost and sit with their lids closed, only looking out occasionally though narrow slits into the bright of the day.

Reptiles and amphibians

In the amphibian eye (of frogs, toads and the like), the lens is huge and almost a perfect sphere, similar to that in a fish eye, and as for most fish, eyesight is not the all-important sense it is in some other groups of animals. Under water the cornea has little refractive power, which is why amphibians and fish have big round lenses to compensate. In such big lenses, accommodation (changing its shape) is not practical so the whole lens is moved backwards or forwards in a rather inefficient attempt to keep the moving image as sharp as possible. The amphibian eye is not brilliant in water, but it is even worse on land. A frog sees moving things better than stationary things, and partly because of conditioning and partly because of eyesight, it could be surrounded by dead flies and starve, although if a moving fly comes into range it is gobbled up right away!

Reptiles, particularly lizards and snakes, have more interesting eyes, but they are built on a similar blueprint, albeit with greater adaption and variation to suit their more diverse habitats.

The glassy stare of a snake can give such an uncomfortable alien feeling as it gazes at you through apparently lidless eyes. Only a snake's eyes are not lidless: each eye has two extremely important lids which are fused together and form a transparent cover. In some cases the transparent cover is formed by only one lid. This cover is called a *spectacle*, which is a rather inappropriate term: the spectacle does not contribute to vision, but protects the eye from damage, so 'safety goggle' might be a more fitting name. Some lizards also have spectacles over their eyes; usually these are the burrowing species that clearly benefit from a transparent outer protective coat. Spectacles arose originally in fish, particularly those that grub around and are bottom feeders such as catfish, but they are at their most 'spectacular' in the snakes.

The chameleon, a lizard famous for its colour-changing act, is equally odd with regard to its eyes. It is the only species which can manage to have one eye pointing forward and the other pointing back at the same time. The eyes are out on 'turrets' on the sides of the chameleon's relatively small head. When exploring the environment the chameleon is still and its eyes swivel around independently, but if it locates potential food, then the eyes come back into line with each other. It needs both eyes to converge on its prey so that it can judge distance and capture its victim with a dart of an impressively long tongue.

The horned lizard has no particularly extraordinary visual capabilities, having rather poor vision and catching and eating its food with its eyes tightly shut. It only eats ants and its thick skin makes it immune to their bites; the only vulnerable part of its body is the eye, hence it has to keep its eyes closed. With its knobbly skin it might not look an inviting meal, but coyotes and other large carnivores sometimes are too hungry to be choosy. If a predator picks on the horned lizard as a potential meal, however, it does it only once. A thick skin is not the lizard's only defence: it also has a very impressive wink. When the lizard winks it squirts blood from a pouch under its lower lid. This blood is mixed with nasty chemicals and, when fired accurately into its attacker's face, is more than enough to deter the hungriest of carnivores.

A truly remarkable lizard called Sphenodon lives on islands off the coast of New Zealand. I spent a long time in a zoo in New Zealand waiting to see this little animal, in vain because it is very shy. I am told that at first glance it looks just like any other lizard. Certainly its conventional eyes are nothing to write home about, but it does have something rather special in that it has a partly functional third eye on the top of its head. This third eye is situated above the *pineal gland* and has a lens and a retina of sorts. Functionally it can distinguish light from dark, but little else is known about what this strange additional eye can do.

Fish

Fish are so varied that it is difficult to generalize and their faculties range from modest vision in the shark-like fish, which have only rods in their retinas, to reasonably good cone/rod vision in the more advanced fish. Sharks rely more on their sense of smell, which can be remarkably sensitive, and on their lateral line system. The lateral line is a row of receptors down the side of a fish which pick up vibrations through the water. A shark, for example, uses its lateral line receptors to pick up the thrashing of a seal or fish in trouble on the surface of the water. Unfortunately for humans that series of vibrations is remarkably like those of a swimmer. The shark, however, is never confused by the smell of blood, which it can pick up at exceptional distances.

Eyesight may be of lesser importance when compared with other senses in many fish, but there are some spectacular exceptions. A South American freshwater fish swims with half of its eye above water and half below. Each eye is divided neatly in two like a figure of eight, with an aerial-type optical system in the upper half and an aquatic-type in the lower half. Aerial and aquatic visual information hit different parts of the retina at the same time.

How does the fish's brain cope? Another oddity is the archer fish. These fish live in muddy rivers and although they swim under the water they somehow manage, with pinpoint accuracy, to spit a stream of water at insects on the leaves of overhanging trees, bringing them down into the river. What kind of eye-to-brain programming is needed to achieve such complex trajectories, which overcome the poor visibility in the water, refraction at the surface, glare from the sun, and still hit small targets? Think back to the last time you were under water in a swimming pool, looking out at the wavy bodies at the pool edge. Even if you wear swimming goggles as an aid, the distortion is considerable.

Surprisingly sight is of considerable importance to many deep-sea fish. As there is little or no light at depth in the ocean, what can the eyes be used for? These deep-sea fish have very sensitive retinas packed with rods; some species have over 25 million receptors per square millimetre. It doesn't make sense until you remember that most, if not all, the animals in the deep glow in the dark, due to luminescence. The eyes of the deep-sea fish are tuned in to picking up the faint glow emitted by a potential mate, possible food or even a predator to be avoided. The deep-sea angler fish has a tentacle sticking out from the front of its head with a luminescent tip. It waves the tentacle about like a fishing rod so that the glowing tip

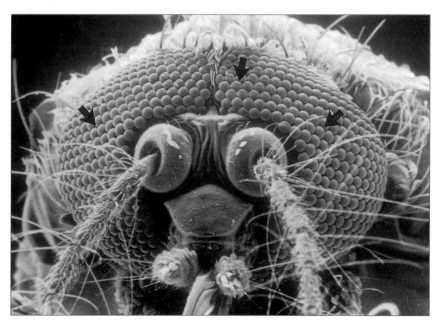

Figure 2.6 The compound eyes (arrows) of a mosquito as seen under the electron microscope. The mosquito does not have a particularly well-developed visual system, but the myriad little eyes which make up its compound eyes seem to cover much of the head. (*Provided by Peter Young, School of Tropical Medicine, Liverpool*)

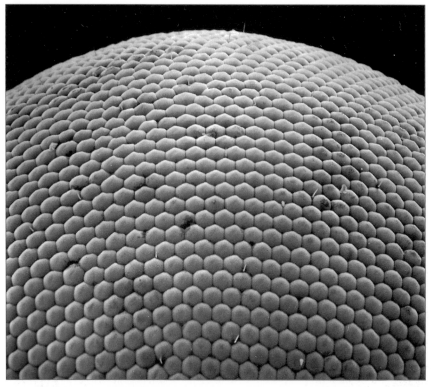

Figure 2.7 Part of the even larger compound eye of a house fly.
(*Provided by Dr Paul Appleton, St Paul's Eye Unit, Liverpool*)

looks like a bug. Other fish locate the glow in the darkness of the deep, but unfortunately their eyes let them down because they don't see the rows of sharp angler-fish teeth lurking behind the 'bug'.

Insects

The *compound eye* of insects such as flies, bees and beetles is a beautiful dome-like structure built of large numbers of tubular units (Figures 2.6 and 2.7). Each of the tubes is an eye in its own right, consisting of a clear outer cover (the cornea), a lens and some photoreceptor or light-sensitive cells to convert light into visual signals. There are two different designs of compound eyes: a daylight and a night-time eye. In the daylight eye each tube is surrounded by opaque pigment so that no light can stray internally between tubes. Insulation gives better acuity, so this is the eye of wasps, bees and butterflies. The night-time eye, found in moths and the like, has no opaque pigment cover so that light does stray between the various tubes. The night design makes best use of what light is available but creates a poor image.

At one time it was thought that in the daytime compound eye, each tube formed an image of only a small part of the view observed by the insect, rather like the bank of television screens sometimes seen at important events where together the screens form a scene but each one only shows a small part of that scene. Alternatively others have suggested that each tube images most of the scene so the insect has many views of the same thing. Biologists are still far from fully understanding the complexities of the beautiful compound eye of the insect.

Beautiful it may be, but does the compound eye function well as a visual organ? The answer is that we don't know, but the best guess is that it is poor in many insects, not bad in some and really quite good in those with the best daylight eyes. Each tube of the compound eye produces a poor image so it is a case of the more tubes the insect has, the better is its eyesight. An ant has only a few tubes in its eye and probably can't see much at all, whereas the kings of the compound eyes are the dragonflies, which can have as many as 30,000 tubes making up each eye. Dragonflies are fast-flying predators that need good vision to catch their food, but there are other insects with vision that is almost as good to help them locate their food, and these include flies, butterflies, beetles and bees.

If eyesight with colour vision were not an important sense to the flies, butterflies and bees, the world would be far less vibrant than it is. Flying insects were around before but came to particular prominence in the Cretaceous period, over 100 million years ago, and at about the same time as flowering plants. Until then pollination of plants had depended mostly on the wind, as it still does for the grasses and many of the trees. The flowering plants produced a source of food for the insects in the form of nectar and edible pollen, and in turn the insects carried the pollen from plant to plant and fertilized them. The problem for the plants was how to advertise their wares and attract the insects to them. This was solved by developing colourful petals and perfume. The flower to humans is a thing of beauty, to an insect it is a source of nourishment and to the plant itself it is just like an advertising hoarding for a fast-food outlet!

It is hard to think of how the world might be if sight was not an important sense to the pollinating insects. Would the Earth just have grasses and some trees, or would the flowers be plain and just give out an intense smell? Maybe the strong smell would not even be a nice one to humans, which is the case with some flowers that depend on nocturnal moths for pollination.

The insect's colour vision is not the same as a human's and it seems that, for example in bees (which have been most studied), they see shorter wavelengths of light than humans. Insects see ultraviolet but, apart from some of the butterflies, most do not see red as anything but black. The inescapable fact is that the colourful flowers that attract us are at least as vibrant to insects, but the insects often see them robed in quite a different gown. White flowers to a bee are bluey-green; yellow and blue petals are particularly attractive to them because, for a bee, they are both primary colours. The bee does not see red but does not see the red poppy as black. The poppy's petals reflect ultraviolet so to a bee the poppy is a brilliant purple. Many flowers look quite different when they are photographed in ultraviolet, having complex lines and patterns that we don't appreciate with our vision but which are revealed in all their glory to the eyes of flying insects.

Other animals

The compound eye is not exclusive to insects, and both the daylight and night-time varieties are to be found in crabs, lobsters, shrimps and even in some specialized worms and snails. In various species of crab, the pigment outside the rods can migrate so that the compound eye can change from the daylight to the night-time version when appropriate. During the day, when dazzle could be a problem, the pigment spreads out, almost like a curtain closing, with the aim of absorbing stray light. At night, when the rods need all the light they can get, the pigment is compacted together. Other animals such as spiders, shellfish, slugs and most snails have simple eyes; the simple eyes sometimes have a lens but often do not, and may be little more than a collection of photoreceptors in a pit. The barnacle has three simple eyes without lenses; they merely react to shadows of passing objects, but passing objects may be predators.

There is one group of animals with superb eyesight which, as yet, we have not mentioned and these are the octopuses and squids. If humans and some of the birds have the best eyesight out of water, the octopus and squid have by far the best eyesight in the water. The squid is a fast hunter-killer which preys on small fish but it, in turn, is the prey of larger animals, including humans. It has amazingly good eyesight which allows it to dart into a shoal and grasp one specific fish which it has locked onto. Shoaling is a defensive formation by which small fish protect themselves during daylight; it bewilders predatory fish but it is no problem for the squid with its superb eyesight and spot-on visual acuity. The octopus is much slower and lives in and around rocks or coral, but it is also a predator living on crabs and similar food. Its victims live in crevices hidden from others, but the octopus can see right into these recesses and prises the crabs out with its long tentacles.

The eyes of the squid and octopus have same features in common with human eyes, for example each one has a lens whose shape can be changed by the action of muscles so the eye can focus on near and far objects. However, the retina on to which the light is focused has photoreceptors on the front rather than at the back, as is the case in humans, this design problem being avoided in these animals, and the receptor cells are more like those found in the compound eye than the rods and cones in mammals. A good eye design is complemented by a highly developed brain, which is particularly large in the areas associated with integrating and co-ordinating visual information. The squid and octopus in their own way are formidable hunter-killers, superbly aided by very effective vision.

FACTS AND OLD WIVES' TALES

✧ It is true that in fading light, our ability to see colour goes, but we seem to be more sensitive to short (blues and greens) than long wavelengths (reds) in dim lighting and so the former remain with us longer. If you are in a garden as dusk is setting in, red and then orange flowers will soon appear black but their stems will remain green. Blue will remain clear for a while and even become more vibrant (towards the ultraviolet).

✧ It is frequently said that holding a book too close to the eyes can be harmful, especially in children. Children often hold books very close to their eyes because they have something that older people have lost – good accommodation (see earlier in this chapter). For them, even very close objects are not blurred. Holding a book close to does no harm to children.

✧ If you want to check how important binocular vision is, try picking blackberries with one eye closed. Be careful not to get too many scratches!

✧ At steeplechases and other jumping races, such as the Grand National, some jockeys show their mount the first fence before the race begins, 'so it can have a good look'. Since a horse has its eyes at the side of its head, it probably does not see much of the fence when it is close to and about to jump. This may be just as well in the case of fences like 'the Chair' and 'Beecher's Brook', but the jockeys are not so fortunate.

Chapter 3

Eye care
Eye care through history, and eye care professionals today

This chapter starts with a short history of eye care through the centuries, then discusses the eye care professionals of today – from oculists to ophthalmologists, what they do and the equipment they use. It will cover both mainstream eye care and alternative therapies.

HISTORICAL EYES: EYE CARE THROUGHOUT HISTORY

Clearly our eyes are most important to our well-being and survival so it comes as no surprise that most of us consider vision to be the most important of the senses and have an utter dread of anything going wrong with our sight. This is the case now and it has been the case throughout most of recorded history. In many cultures the eye doctor, once called an *oculist* and now called an *ophthalmologist*, has had a prestigious place in society and has been treated with a special kind of reverence. The reverence has been earned by saving sight. Often in the past that precious commodity has been squandered through quackery and ignorance, but ophthalmology also has thousands of years of spectacular successes. After all there is nothing more effective in a doctor's repertoire than to restore some sight to a blind cataract patient by a relatively simple needling procedure.

China and India

The first eye specialists or oculists were associated with the relatively sophisticated civilizations of ancient China. Unfortunately little is known of their techniques, treatments or surgery. It is known only that the healers were treated with great respect and applied a mixture of approaches including faith healing, demonology, herbalism and very sophisticated forms of acupuncture.

The eye surgeons of ancient India no doubt took much of their learning from China, but also made great advances in their own right, particularly in the surgical treatment of cataract. Cataract was (and still is) rampant in the Indian subcontinent and the early operation of *couching* was refined there. This involved using a lancet or needle to push the opaque, cataractous lens out of the visual plane.

Babylon

Eye specialists were prominent in the Sumerian Empire and, as with other types of doctor during the period, their treatments relied on appeasing the gods, hocus-pocus, herbal medicine and some surgery. Sumeria gave way to other empires in the same region, culminating in Babylonia. Written information is available from this period in the form of a code of practice which dates back to almost 2000 BC. The code states that if a doctor 'operates on the eye with a copper lancet, [he] shall charge 10 shekels of silver'. This would have been a great deal of money in Babylonian society and a few successful operations could make the surgeon very rich. On the down side, the code went on to state that if the operation was unsuccessful the surgeon's hands might be cut off!

Medical treatment of eye problems usually involved the reading of omens and defeating the power of demons. Chanting to Ea, the powerful god of the waters, was also thought to be valuable. However, on a more practical level, sensible use of bandaging and the availability of an impressive range of herbs and minerals would guarantee some happy customers, although several treatments left much to be desired. One example is dryness of the eye, which could be treated by oils or, if you chose the wrong doctor, the insides of a yellow frog. Or for soreness of the eye, the recommended treatment was bathing it with the urine of a white dog.

Egypt

Eye medicine was listed as being one of the main specialities of the medicine of ancient Egypt. Writings from around 1500 BC, however, show that, although in other branches of medicine the Egyptians may have been progressive, ophthalmology was not at the front of the queue. An example of a general 'cure all' treatment for a number of eye problems was to pulverize human brains in honey to make a paste and then cover the eye with the mess. In Egypt all manner of pastes were made to apply on and around the eyes, and these eye pastes were used for thousands of years. A black paste containing antimony was particularly popular and was applied on the brows and the lids. Originally it was to ward off infection but, as it made the eyes appear more striking, it soon came into regular use as a cosmetic (see chapter 6).

Greece

Turning to the medicine of Classical Greece, the first name to be mentioned must be that of Hippocrates (*c.* 460–375 BC), the father of medicine and from whom the concept of the Hippocratic Oath comes. In his writings he mentions a number of eye diseases, although it must be said that the Greek physicians didn't really have a good working knowledge of ocular structure and function. They thought, for example, that the inside of the eye was all jelly (vitreous) and when it cooled down it became solid (the lens). The lack of a clear appreciation of ocular anatomy and function, however, did not stop the Greek physicians from having a good clinical awareness. They had a profound influence on medicine and, in turn, on ophthalmology throughout the following centuries.

Living in a dry and hot country, the Greeks were competent on the diagnosis of ocular inflammations of various types which they called 'ophthalmia'. Epidemics of *red eye* (inflammation of the eye) were all too common in the Mediterranean countries. Other examples of terminology introduced by the ancient Greeks include *'amblyopia'* for a loss of visual function and 'glaukos', for what we now term *glaucoma* (see chapter 4). Glaukos was a watery blue colour describing the appearance of an eye with advanced glaucoma. *Squint* was recognized and also it was known that the children of squinting parents were highly likely to have a squint themselves. The technical term for squint is *strabismus* – a Greek word. Such was the influence of Hippocrates on future medicine that the language of medicine is predominantly Greek.

Rome

Latin also has its place in the language of medicine because of highly influential Roman doctors such as Galen (*c.* AD 130–200) (probably, in fact, a Greek by birth). Much of their original knowledge came after the incorporation of Greece into the Roman Empire, but new ideas and treatments came from the many other parts of their domain. The cataract operation of couching was an important part of Roman surgery and was probably introduced through contact with the East. However, Galen in one of his books claimed that the cataract operation was discovered by watching goats. It was affirmed that if a goat had a cataract it pricked its eye on a thorn bush! Eye medications called *collyrias* were a common form of treatment, as were frequent bleedings and laxatives. The medicinal value of wine was also well appreciated, and probably very necessary after some of the former treatments.

It has been an oft-reported tale that Romans sometimes used jewels to see distance. The most famous short-sighted Roman was Nero who is reputed to have watched Christians being eaten by lions and gladiator fights in the arena through a very large emerald. A more useful magnifying agent was a thin glass goblet filled with water, which was used by ageing Roman academics as a reading aid.

Arabia

During the so-called dark ages after the fall of Rome and through the Middle Ages, medical knowledge in Europe declined to nothing, but the Graeco-Roman tradition was safeguarded by Arabian doctors through these times and beyond. They made significant advances in their own right, including a suction procedure for the surgical treatment of soft cataracts and surgical treatments for early *trachoma* (see chapter 4). It was in this environment that the earliest advances in the understanding of the science of optics were made. Alhazen who lived in the tenth century conducted some of the first scientific works on the magnifying power of lenses.

Medieval Europe

In the Middle Ages in Europe, medicine was primitive and eye care in particular was in disrepute. The people who looked at eyes were quack oculists who went on their way to the next village before their bogus cures could be found out. The 'wise women' of a community would also contribute what they could but much of medicine, including ophthalmology, was no longer a suitable subject for intelligent pursuit. After all, the medieval Church dictated that illness could be cured by faith, and this tended to stifle any other avenues of care. This was the time of holy relics and people with anything wrong with their eyes or who were blind visited a shrine which had a relic of an appropriate saint. There were many saints and many relics associated with such an emotive condition as blindness, but the relics were likely to be as bogus as the itinerant oculists.

Eventually centres of medical learning such as Montpellier in France and Salerno in Italy did became established, but eye operations were very much the province of the untrained even when surgery and medicine were becoming re-established. Couching of cataracts for example was undertaken by the barber-surgeons and was an operation thought to be inappropriate for medical people trained in universities and centres of learning. Not all the wise women, barber-surgeons and oculists were incompetent, but those with talent were so rare that their deeds became legendary. Trotula, who did everything from managing births to eye surgery, is depicted as Dame Trot in early plays and old nursery rhymes.

When translations of Arabic texts such as those of Alhazen became available in Europe, they stimulated a new interest in vision and optics. One of the most prominent authorities of the time was Roger Bacon (1214–94) who is thought by some to be the inventor of eye glasses, but there are other medieval monks with an equally good or poor claim. In a Florentine graveyard there is an inscription on a grave which says: 'Here lies Salvino d'Armato of the Armati of Florence, inventor of spectacles.' It continues: 'May God forgive him his sins AD 1317', perhaps an unfortunate association of phrases. It does, however, seem that spectacles existed in Europe around the end of the thirteenth century. They were also seen by Marco Polo on his travels in China, so they are thought to have been first made there around the same time as in Europe. The first lenses for eye glasses were probably made of quartz rather than glass.

Through to the present day

During the Renaissance there was a new vitality in science and medicine which had a spill over to ophthalmology. A better understanding of eye function and diseases resulted. Leonardo da Vinci was among several who made accurate drawings of the eye, the optic nerve and their relation to the brain. The outstanding ophthalmologist of the time was Georg Bartisch (1535–1606) who is justifiably considered to be the founder of modern ophthalmology. The true basis of cataract formation began to be understood and gradually cataract treatment became the business of proper surgeons and not the barber-surgeons or poorly trained oculists. The watershed was the invention by Jacques Daviel in 1750 of a cataract operation which was technically far more difficult than couching or needling (pushing the lens out of the way of light entering the eye) and involved the removal of the opaque lens from the eye. Daviel was subjected to much professional abuse because many of the oculists of that time were not sufficiently skilful and often botched the more complex surgery required, but as time went by and more good surgeons did the procedure, lens removal became a very successful operation.

Eye glasses (Figure 3.1) came into more common use, although buying these was an expensive business (even more so than today) and simply a matter of trying on what was available and seeing which best suited your needs. Glasses became a fad in eighteenth-century Europe when it was very fashionable to be seen with them. Eye glasses do nothing to weaken eyes, being only an aid to poor vision (see later in this chapter for more on this subject), but oculists, and popular opinion, right through to the beginning of the twentieth century have been either hostile to glasses or ambivalent. Holding on to this myth has done a disservice to the poor sighted.

The first hospital dedicated to eye treatment and teaching was established in 1786 by Georg Beer in Austria. In London, Moorfields Eye Hospital was founded in 1805 to cope with the massive increase in eye problems which had arisen following the return of troops from Egypt. Soldiers and sailors returned with numerous infectious eye diseases like trachoma and

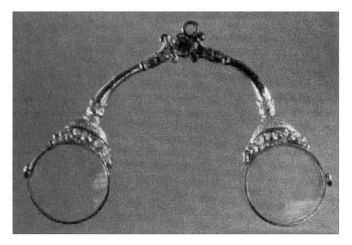

Figure 3.1 Scissor spectacles from around 1750.
(*Source*: *Journal of Ophthalmology* (103: 1110, 1997), courtesy of the
Museum of Ophthalmology, Foundation of the American Academy of
Ophthalmology, San Francisco, California)

spread them through the population. Other institutions followed around the world and ophthalmology began to be seen as a respectable branch of medicine, although there were still oculists such as Chevalier Taylor (1703–72), who blinded Bach (see chapter 5), to hold the speciality back.

Another factor holding back advances in ophthalmology was a purely technical one: there were insufficient technical aids with which to examine such a small, delicate and complex structure. The invention of the *ophthalmoscope* in 1851 by Helmholtz was a giant step forward into the modern age.

Spectacle frames were first made of paper, leather or even wood and must have been very uncomfortable. Surprisingly it was not until well into the eighteenth century that someone had the bright idea of keeping spectacles in place with 'legs' going behind the ear. Although near lenses were available from the thirteenth century, it wasn't until the sixteenth century that distance lenses were made. Putting the two together took until the end of the eighteenth century and one of those involved in making double spectacles or *bifocals* was Benjamin Franklin, the famous American statesman and scientist.

Contact lenses seem a very modern idea so it is perhaps surprising that they were thought of first in Renaissance Italy. It may be less of a surprise to hear that they were yet another brainchild of Leonardo da Vinci. Following a few false starts, the first practical effort was glass contact lenses created by Adolph Fick and Ernst Abbe in Germany in 1888. Hard plastic lenses for limited wear came from Teissler in 1937. Since this time the lenses have become thinner and more biologically acceptable to the eye, and huge progress has been made with the wide range of soft lenses introduced in recent years.

EYE PROFESSIONALS

Eye care has come from modest beginnings, through a chequered history of itinerant oculists and hocus-pocus to the exact and demanding discipline it is today. Eye care requires a wide range of skills and 'state-of-the-art machinery', so the discipline is shared by a range of different professionals, each with their own training and expertise, working together to provide a full range of services. The trouble is that it is not always clear to the general public what each of these experts does and how they relate outside and inside an eye department.

I was most impressed with an article written by Dr Ann Robertson in the health section of the 14th January 1997 edition of the *Independent.* Dr Robertson outlined very effectively a journey of confusion and bewilderment which started when she and her husband first noticed that their four-year-old son might have a squint. None of the health professionals mentioned in this article come across as being either easy to understand or able to communicate terribly well to the concerned parents exactly what it is they do. Dr Robertson is a general practitioner and, if she found the people and the system difficult to grasp, what chance has anyone else?

Consultant ophthalmologist

An *ophthalmologist* is a specialist eye doctor who is trained as both a physician and a surgeon. Since ophthalmologists are surgeons they hold the title Mr or Ms, rather than Dr, in common with general surgeons and harking back to their barber-surgeon origins.*

Ophthalmologists train in all aspects of eye care and can provide a complete service. However, it is usual, particularly in university departments, for the consultants to sub-specialize in a particular area of ophthalmology. Each consultant has general and speciality clinics, so even within ophthalmology itself there are divisions of proficiency. There are fewer than 700 consultant eye doctors in Britain, which is an extremely low number compared with other European countries and the USA. Part of the reason

---

* It should be said, however, that only one in ten patients who go to an eye hospital need surgery. Most of the ophthalmologist's work is as a physician, so please don't think that because you have an appointment in the hospital eye department that means that someone is going to operate on your eyes. Eye operations are a small part of the activities of an eye department.

for this is because elsewhere ophthalmologists do eye tests for routine prescription of glasses, whereas in Britain this job is done by the optometrist.

Junior eye doctor

As with any other part of the hospital system, a doctor who wants to specialize in ophthalmology has to pass professional exams and then undergo an extensive training programme. A graduate from medical school takes a number of temporary jobs in hospitals where he or she gains further training and uses his or her developing skills.

The doctor keen to move into ophthalmology will obtain training and experience in senior house officer (SHO) posts in this speciality in different parts of the country. After a variable period, probably not less than three years, and when the professional exams have been passed the SHO will apply for a training position in one of the university training regions.

The successful applicant will then spend a further four to four and a half years rotating between consultant 'firms' (consultants' support teams of junior doctors) to gain the broadest possible experience. Further time may be spent in research fellowships or in highly specialized clinical fellowships before applying for a consultancy post. The traditional term for these doctors is 'registrar' (which is to be phased out) but don't think of them as being 'wet behind the ears': they have undergone a long training schedule before they ever see you.

General practitioner

General practitioners (GPs) are the front line of health care. If you have something wrong with your eye, as with any other part of you, you go and see your local GP. As a rule GPs are not strong on eye problems because during their lengthy medical training they spend only a few weeks doing ophthalmology. However, if your eye problem requires it, your GP will get you a hospital appointment to see a specialist. Of course, you can go directly to an eye unit's accident and emergency department for an acute problem, but a GP letter is the usual route by which to see an ophthalmologist.

Some GPs have a special interest in ophthalmology and go back to hospital for additional training. A number of the bigger practices now have speciality GPs, one of whom may be for eye problems; they will be on hand for specialist opinion on first-time patients, but will also be involved in the long-term care of patients with a chronic eye problem that needs periodic monitoring.

Optometrist and optician

The *optometrist* has three main roles in the community. The first is to conduct eye tests and check vision for an appropriate prescription, the second is to sell glasses and contact lenses, but the third can be the most important and that is to check for some of the more common eye diseases. Although optometrists are not doctors they have a key position in the chain of vision health care. Indeed, for some eye conditions like glaucoma they are the front-line defence; the vast majority of suspected glaucoma sufferers come to the hospital because their optometrist has picked up tell-tale signs. If the optometrist during the eye test suspects an eye problem, the patient is sent to his or her GP for referral on to an eye department. Optometrists would like to refer directly to hospital eye departments, arguing that this will speed things up, but GPs contend that they are a necessary link in the chain to prevent over-referring. At present some hospitals and health regions do accept direct optometrist referrals but this is not universal.

What is the difference between an optometrist and an *optician*? The answer is that essentially they are one and the same. At one time the profession was not degree-based and all those who passed the professional exams were licensed opticians. Opticians refracted and dispensed spectacles (dispensing opticians), but progressively they became more involved in screening for eye disease (ophthalmic opticians). Much of the new development coincided with the requirement to have a BSc degree before gaining practical experience and then sitting the professional exams, and also around this time contact lens wearing became more popular. Clearly the role of the high street optician had evolved into something far broader than in the past, so many ophthalmic opticians prefer to use the American term 'optometrist' to highlight their increased responsibilities.

The vast majority of British GPs have had only a rudimentary ophthalmic experience and training, and the numbers of ophthalmologists are low. This means that there is a place for a group of health professionals in the front line of eye care. It is the expectation of many optometrists that increasingly they will take up this role. Not only do they see themselves diagnosing common eye diseases in people who come for eye tests, but also they wish to prescribe eye drops for minor ailments and to undertake some of the routine check-ups on hospital-diagnosed patients with chronic but stable ocular conditions, for example some long-term glaucoma patients.

Such an expansion in the optometrist's role is merely a matter of debate at present. There are concerns expressed both by ophthalmologists and by GPs that medicine should not be taken out of the control of qualified doctors and put into the hands of other professionals. All this may lie in the future, but with increasing demands on the health service the expanding role of the optometrists in primary health care is seen as an attractive option in some quarters. Not all optometrists work from the high street; hospital eye departments also include optometrists. Optometrists in hospitals prescribe glasses and contact lenses for patients with visual disabilities as a consequence of eye disease. They work hand-in-hand with the ophthalmologists to make the very best of what vision is left after the eye problem has been addressed.

University courses for a degree in optometry and/or visual sciences are available at the City University, London; University of Wales, Cardiff; Aston University, Birmingham; UMIST, Manchester; Bradford University; Caledonian University, Glasgow; Anglia Polytechnic University, Cambridge; and University of Ulster, Coleraine.

Orthoptist

Orthoptists are vision professionals and their job is to investigate, diagnose and treat disorders of eye movement, binocular vision and other problems of this type. Orthoptists usually are based in hospital eye departments but increasingly they are involved in the community. Although the modern orthoptist now works extensively with adults who have problems with eye movement as a result of injury and such like, the traditional role is in working with children suffering from different types of squints (see chapter 4 for more on squint). Squints in children are best treated when they are picked up early, so it is now common practice for orthoptists to go into nursery and primary schools and screen for squint and related conditions.

The profession is an evolving one and many orthoptists are involved with patient care away from their traditional areas of expertise. It is not unusual to find orthoptists involved in clinics concerned with the diagnosis and treatment of glaucoma. Orthoptists can find a role in rehabilitation of patients with facial paralysis or in the recovery of stroke patients. It is a specialized job requiring considerable skills so, since the beginning of the 1990s, new orthoptists have been required to gain an orthoptics BSc degree at university before pursuing their professional qualifications.

Degree courses in orthoptics are available at the University of Liverpool and the University of Sheffield.

Eye nurse

Nurses have a general training in all branches of health care, but there are opportunities to specialize and become involved in one or more areas of patient provision, such as midwifery, psychiatric medicine or ophthalmology. A nurse's training equips him or her to deal with hospital activities in all branches of medicine, but those based in eye departments need additional on-site training to be familiar with eye conditions which present in accident and emergency, the complex equipment used for eye assessment in clinics, and the microsurgery procedures specific to ocular operating theatres. A nurse who specializes in an aspect of eye care is often called an *eye nurse practitioner* (Figure 3.2).

Not all eye nurse practitioners work in a hospital setting. In some regions

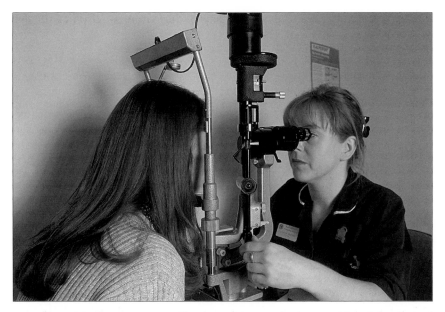

Figure 3.2 An eye nurse practitioner examining a patient's eyes with a slit lamp.

there are community nurses with eye training. Their role is multiple: they check between hospital visits on patients who have just had eye operations, they provide home support for those with chronic eye problems, they can be involved in school or community screening programmes to identify early eye problems and in addition they provide support, information and advice for the recently blind and partially sighted.

Social worker

There are hospital social workers who have specific expertise in the problems of the visually handicapped. Their role complements and bolsters that of the other eye health professionals by making the quality of life of those who are temporarily or permanently visually handicapped substantially better. They provide counselling when needed, advice on social and financial support if required, and a friendly shoulder to lean on at all times.

Eye support technician

In the modern eye department there is a large amount of complex equipment, ranging from computers to lasers, which is needed for the examination of the eye or for treating eye conditions. Some departments have 'in-house' technicians to maintain or even run some of the equipment in clinics, examination rooms and theatres. Virtually all eye departments have photographic technicians who specialize in taking routine reference photographs of patients' eyes. They may be involved in taking pictures of the inside of the eye using some of the more complex photographic equipment and certainly they would process the resultant films for later interpretation by the doctors. A highly specialized job undertaken by some technicians is making, colouring and matching artificial eyes – an uncommon, but highly skilled profession.

Oculist

Oculist is an all-encompassing term which covers anyone who works with eye diseases or weaknesses of the eye. It is an old word often associated with the charlatan, roaming eye doctors of the past, who knew little and talked a lot, already discussed in this chapter. If you called any eye professional an oculist you would be dictionary-accurate, but they might not like it.

ALTERNATIVE EYES

I must admit to having a very limited knowledge of alternative medicine so for those with a particular interest, I would recommend that you look at more informed literature (see Further Reading). The two aspects of alternative medicine I wish to cover are iridology, whose practitioners consider that they can diagnose illness in the body from patterns in the iris, and the views of those who suggest eye exercises as an alternative to glasses.

Iridology in complementary medicine

The iris gives the eye its colour (see chapter 1) but, if it is looked at closely with a magnifying lens, it can be seen that the front surface of the iris is not uniform either in colour or in markings. The iris surface has folds, pits, craters, freckles and sometimes *naevi* (larger freckles), and other irregularities which make it anything but smooth. Every person's eye markings are unique to them, like a fingerprint.

To the anatomist and ophthalmologist the irregularities are just anatomic variables of minor interest (except on rare occasions when a *melanoma* cancer develops on the iris surface), but to one group of alternative therapists called *iridologists* the surface features and colour characteristics are a map which they believe provides information about the past and present health of the patients that they examine. Iridologists are not just concerned with the health of the eye, although this is of interest to them also; they use the features of the iris to chart existing and potential health problems throughout the body. To quote James and Sheelagh Colton, who are authorities publishing and practising in the field, iridologists believe that 'The iris displays our individual blueprint of inherent strengths and weaknesses.'

This does not mean that if someone develops a pain in the stomach a blotch will form on the iris which will disappear when the trouble is relieved. However, an iridologist would look in the region of the iris associated with the stomach (stomach and bowels are said to be located around the pupil, see Plate 8) and may find markings there that they would associate with hereditary weakness.

Iridology was first practised by a Hungarian doctor called von Peczely (1822–1911) who proposed that illness could be diagnosed from examination of the iris. Iridology was then and still is considered highly dubious by many in the medical professions. Peczely's iridial maps and teachings survived, and have become adapted over the years to those used by the practitioners of today. It is believed by iridologists that, among other things, people with brown eyes are prone to blood-related problems, green-eyed people tend to have liver problems and those with blue eyes are more likely to suffer from respiratory disease and rheumatism.

The iris map can be divided into territories and is followed like a 60-minute clock. Taking the right iris, at around 0 minutes (or 12 o'clock) is the region which relates to the brain, at 20 minutes is the bladder, at 30 minutes the kidney, and between 45 and 50 minutes is the lung. Around the pupil are the stomach and bowels, whereas the heart lies in territories on the outside right and left. The left eye is not quite the mirror image, e.g. the lung region in the left is between 10 and 15 minutes, but the mirror position of the liver area is held by the spleen. Plate 8 is a simplified version of a minute amount of the information that is contained in 'The British Iris Chart' (obtainable from the British Society of Iridologists, whose address is given at the end of this book).

I have an on-going research interest in the iris and I do not know if there is any substance to the iridologists' claims that the iris is a diagnostic map by which human illness can be determined. At present, however, the iris still has many secrets for the scientists to unravel. While some doctors do practise iridology, therapists need not have a medical degree or, for that matter, any formal training as health professionals. Diagnosis of human disease, irrespective of what procedure is used, should be undertaken by or in conjunction with medical practitioners; anything else may be unsafe. Iridology is described by its adherents as being a safe and valuable diagnostic tool. The examination may be harmless but it is only safe if it doesn't divert a patient with a serious medical problem from conventional treatment. If you attend an iridologist and he or she suspects you have a problem, make sure you also get some conventional wisdom from your GP to complement that opinion. Iridology may have diagnostic value but I know of no ophthalmologist who holds that view at present.

Exercises for eyes as an alternative to glasses

Basic ophthalmic and optometric opinion is that eye exercises (other than those given by orthoptists – see earlier), while doing nothing untoward, do not do what they claim, namely (a) to prevent the need for glasses if you don't wear them already; (b) to improve your eyesight such that you might no longer need your glasses, or at least to reduce the correction; and even, (c) to prevent the development of certain eye diseases, an example being cataract, and childhood visual problems such as squint.

Those who advocate eyesight improvement by exercise frequently follow the teachings of W. H. Bates who was a firm champion of the view that short sight and long sight have little to do with the size of the eyeball (the conventional opinion of nearly all ophthalmologists), but are caused by a problem of the extraocular muscles (see chapters 1 and 2). He argued that the muscles can be retrained so that the visual problem is corrected. In addition he put forward his opinion that to have good vision you also need to have good general health, emotional stability and mental well-being. His theories gain much support from those in alternative medicine, but are disliked by conventional eye care professionals.

The proposed exercises are varied but combine eye manipulations with the establishment of a stress-free mental state. *Bates therapists* recommend breathing exercises and promote a positive frame of mind. They use eye movement procedures like 'the magic pencil', which involves imagining there is a pencil at the end of your nose and forming the habit of drawing around objects in your field of vision, large ones at first then smaller. The object is to exercise the eyes so that they become more mobile. Another involves balancing an imaginary feather on the end of the nose to gain visual relaxation. Vision is also thought to be improved by drawing mental images.

Palming is another Bates technique and this requires placing the palms of the hands over the eyes and imagining colourful pictures; this is also said by the Bates therapists to relax the eyes. Mandalas are patterns like the ripples in a pond when a stone is thrown into the water, and these plus fan shapes and spirals are used to stimulate the 'liveliness' of the eyes. Bates teachers usually emphasize the importance of the sun for health and recommend exercises whereby the individual sits looking at the sun with eyes closed. This *sunning* procedure, as it is often called, is potentially harmful because if the eyes are inadvertently opened while looking at the sun, the retina or, even worse, the macula can be burnt. Sun-gazing, in any form, is potentially hazardous.

However, apart from sunning, nothing that I have read of the Bates procedures and other alternative eye exercise strategies seems harmful and, in the context of relaxation and the relief of stress, may well do some general good. On the down side, Bates therapists do recommend that those who wear eye glasses or contact lenses, should go back to their optician and get a lesser correction or indeed abandon their glasses altogether. The under-correction means that vision will be poorer than normal, which has safety implications when driving a car, for example. In their defence, they do recommend that people don't correct beneath the minimum legal driving requirement (see later in this chapter) and they also have eye exercises specifically for drivers.

It is worrying that Bates teachers have such a poor opinion of conventional treatment for childhood visual problems, particularly squint (see chapter 4 for details of squint and its conventional treatment). The procedures and exercises conducted by eye doctors and their professional colleagues, the orthoptists, are designed to get the best possible vision in both eyes. If the squinting eye and the good eye don't visually fuse together the child will have double vision. The child's brain overcomes the double vision by suppressing sight in the squinting eye (a condition called *amblyopia*; see also chapter 4). Amblyopia can also develop in a child who doesn't squint but needs a large correction in one eye.

This visual suppression can be overcome by appropriate glasses, exercises, patching the good eye, and surgery, if necessary. However, with time it becomes more difficult to overcome the squint and the amblyopia, and after the child is seven years of age the difficulties increase considerably. It is true that whereas the squint may well be corrected by conventional treatment, sometimes the vision in the *lazy eye* is not quite what is hoped for. However, the level of success that Bates therapists have for their patients by way of comparison is unclear. The worry with regard to the Bates practices for natural treatment of squint, which involve a series of exercises (including a technique called tromboning where a visual target is moved forwards and backwards in the fashion of the slider on a trombone), is that some patients might not receive conventional treatment until it is too late to be of any good.

The conventional view of consultant eye doctors on short- and long-sightedness is that visual weakness is all to do with the size of the eye. A large eye will tend towards short sight, and a small one towards long sight, and these characteristics have much to do with a person's genes: you are born with the characteristics carried by your family. As one consultant, Mr Patrick Trevor-Roper, has put it, 'We can count it as amply established that nothing we can do – no exercises or spectacles, diet or drugs – will have any influence on the ultimate degree of near-sightedness.' This, of course, runs counter to all that the Bates therapists say about better vision through exercise. Both alternative and conventional therapists consider eye exercise as valuable in the treatment of squint, but they come from entirely different standpoints.

A VISIT TO THE HIGH STREET OPTOMETRIST

Have you ever been for an eye check-up? If so, how often do you go to have your eyes tested by an optometrist? More to the point, how often should you go for a check-up? The Royal National Institute for the Blind (RNIB) suggests that everyone should go for an eye test every two years. That certainly should be the case if you are forty, or even slightly younger, because that is when age causes changes in the lens and ciliary body (see chapters 1 and 2) and glasses may well be necessary. Also it is important to remember that many of the most important eye diseases become more common in later life, such as glaucoma, *age-related macular degeneration*, cataract and *diabetic eye disease.*

The eye test

When you go for an eye test with the optometrist (Figure 3.3), you should take with you the names of any medicines you are currently taking, and the name and address of your doctor may also be useful. If you have been for a correction in the past, then any glasses you wear should be taken along as well. The eye test takes not less than 20 minutes and you should expect the appointment to be around 30 minutes in all. If the test is shorter

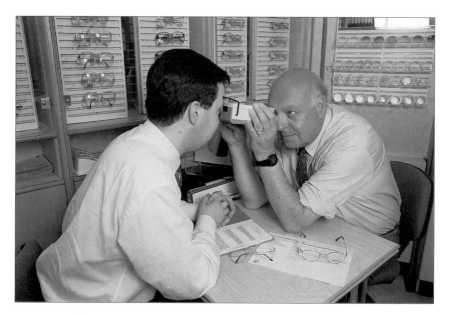

Figure 3.3 An optometrist with a patient.

than 20 minutes, it is worth asking if all the appropriate tests have been done!

You will be asked to read the letters of a chart. The Snellen chart mentioned in chapter 2 consists of different letters of different sizes, and the more rows you read the smaller the letters are. This chart will determine your distance vision. Whether or not you have astigmatism, a visual blurring produced by an irregularity in the surface of the cornea, will be evaluated during the test. At some stage in the test your near vision will also be checked. You will be asked to read from a handbook or pad placed in your normal reading position. The letters of the various passages are of different sizes and the best size at the particular reading distance is judged.

A light will be shone into your eye so that the optometrist can see the front of it and also to make sure that your pupil reacts properly to light. The optometrist will then use a magnifying instrument called an *ophthalmoscope* to look at your lens for cataract (see chapter 4), then at the retina and optic nerve head. People with diabetes can be prone to eye problems related to their disease (see chapter 4), so do make your optician aware if you suffer from diabetes and extra checks can be done.

You will be asked to gaze in different directions to make sure that the eye muscles (the extraocular muscles; see chapter 1) are functioning normally. In addition, many practices routinely check for higher than normal eye pressure, using an instrument which is placed close to, but not on, the front of the eye. All you will feel is a puff of air (Figure 3.4). Higher than normal eye pressure is a feature of the eye condition called glaucoma (for more detail, see chapter 4). Even if you fail this test it doesn't mean you have glaucoma, but it does mean that it will be recommended to your GP that you go to an eye department at a local hospital for a thorough check-up. The optometrist's machine for measuring eye pressure is not as accurate as those used in hospital, so you may find that the actual pressure is not as high as was first suspected. Even if it is found to be high, fewer than half the people with greater than normal eye pressure actually have glaucoma. If you are over 40 years of age and/or you have a member of your family with glaucoma, then you should make sure you get a pressure test as part of your eye check-up.

The next part of the eye test will be to work out your correction if it turns out that you do need glasses. The optometrist will place a series of trial spectacle lenses in front of your eyes and the least powerful lens that will give you the best possible vision (visual acuity; see chapter 2) for each eye will be decided. Also your correction will be done for the reading test if required. Alternatively your correction can be determined using a machine called a *retinoscope* which is an aid to the optometrist to help decide on the ideal lenses for your glasses. Following your test you will be given a

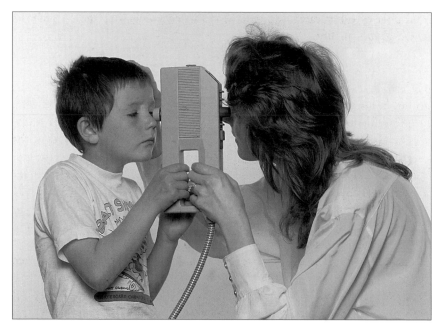

Figure 3.4 Eye pressure measurement.

form describing your vision details and this is a prescription for your glasses or contact lenses. This prescription can be made up by any optometrist using whatever frames or contact lenses you prefer, providing they are suitable for you.

Of course an eye test costs money for many of us, despite the efforts of pressure groups to persuade the government to reinstate free eye tests for all in the UK. Also eye glasses are expensive. Is it really necessary to go for an eye test? Why not just pick up a pair of spectacles from a display in a store? They are cheaper and there is not all that fuss and bother. While there is nothing wrong with trying to get the best price for your glasses, I believe there is a need to visit an optician on a regular basis, especially in the case of older people. The optician, through the eye test, will identify the best possible correction for your eyes; picking glasses from a shelf will only give an approximate correction. Even more important from my point of view is that the risk of eye illnesses becomes greater as we get older (see chapters 4 and 7); the sooner these problems are picked up, the better chance there is of preserving good vision. The high street optometrist is the first line of defence for the health of your eyes.

The National Health Service will pay the cost of the eye test for some groups of people, for example pensioners, people under 16 or on income support, and people over 40 with a relative who has glaucoma. There are a number of other categories so it is worth checking with the optometrist to see if you qualify.

Spectacles

The lenses of spectacles are made of either plastic or glass. The plastic lenses do not last as well and scratch rather easily, but glass lenses are heavier and, in an accident, are far more dangerous. If you do opt for glass lenses be very careful about choosing your frame; if the frame is also heavy, then the weight may be troublesome when you wear your glasses for a long period. I have had my nose broken several times, a legacy of a misspent youth playing rugby and such like, and can't bear the weight of heavy glasses. The most common form of lens is the single vision lens which can be either for reading or for distance (see Figure 3.5). If you want both functions from the one set of spectacles then you require *bifocal lenses* or *varifocal lenses.*

The bifocal lens is simply two different lenses joined together in each eye-piece of your frame. The upper correction is for seeing at distance and the lower section is a reading correction. Bifocals do not suit everyone, but with only a little practice most people soon get used to them. Varifocals also have a distance correction in the upper part of the lens and a reading correction in the lower part, but between the two is a transition zone. Like bifocals, varifocals take a little getting used to: my mother initially proudly sported her new varifocals, but soon gave up on them for regular use. She had difficulty walking down stairs because the stairs seemed too magnified to her, and in addition she found it tiring to keep moving her head when she was reading (the reading lens is of course much smaller than that in normal reading glasses, so it may not be possible to see to the end of a page without turning your head).

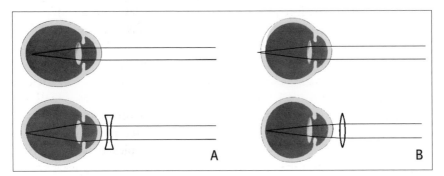

Figure 3.5 (A) Short-sighted people have big eyes and their focusing system brings the light from far objects into sharp focus in front of the retina. (B) Long-sighted people have a focusing system which brings near objects into focus behind the retina. Glasses or contact lenses are needed to make the appropriate correction: for short sight a concave lens and for long sight a convex lens.

Contact lenses

Some people find the weight of glasses uncomfortable; others don't like the restriction of the field of view that glasses bring, whereby side vision is reduced rather like when wearing a hood. Sportspeople often find their glasses an inconvenience or even have to abandon them and cope with weak sight while they play. Some people find glasses unattractive, a stigma which is hardly deserved today given the huge range of styles of frames and lenses available.

An alternative to glasses is contact lenses and these are of two basic types: hard and soft lenses. The hard type are rigid; they are made of several different materials and include gas permeable lenses. Remember that the cornea obtains oxygen and nutrients from the tear film on the surface epithelium of the cornea. The tear film prevents corneal drying and has a general protective role. The insertion of a contact lens is effectively putting a foreign body on to the eye, with the potential to disrupt the delicate balance at the surface of the cornea. The properties of some types of hard lenses are such that they do interfere with the oxygen entry into the cornea. For long-term use gas permeable lenses are recommended because they do not hinder oxygen exchange. They should also have sound surface wetting features so that a good tear film can develop between the lens and the cornea.

Soft lenses are flexible, larger and adhere well, but are more delicate. They are made from polymers which 'like' water so their water content can be as much as 85 per cent. There are a variety of types of soft lens available and these include daily wear lenses, extended wear lenses and, at the other extreme, daily use disposable lenses.

All contact lenses, no matter what type, need to be handled with care and scrupulously looked after. If you are going to handle your lenses, then wash your hands first of all. You can use soft tissue paper to wipe hard lenses but never do this to soft lenses. The cleaning and storage solutions recommended for hard lenses are different from those for soft lenses so don't be tempted to use hard lens solutions on the less robust soft lenses or you will ruin them. Soft lenses are made of a delicate material and are easily scratched, so look out for blemishes and marks on your lenses.

Remember that you risk the health of your eyes if you don't look after your lenses properly and fail to follow the instructions for cleaning and maintaining them. Over the years that I have spent working in eye pathology departments, there has been a steady increase in severe eye problems associated with contact lens wear. Contact lenses are a valuable development that gives options beyond glasses, but they cannot be treated as casually as many of us treat our glasses. Contact lenses are in intimate contact with a very vulnerable part of the body and in the worst circumstances can breach the natural defences of the eye (see chapter 1) and give invading germs a helping hand.

Eyes and lenses need to be treated carefully and with respect, and contact lenses can prove an invaluable aid to vision. I think that daily wear lenses are best suited to meticulous well-organized people. This does not describe me so I would opt for daily use disposables if I wanted contact lenses. However, experts on the various types of contact lenses have told me that disposable lenses come top of the list for infection problems. This may be because users do not always adhere to the instructions and dispose of their lenses when they should. There are advantages and disadvantages with each type of lens, so make sure you know what they are when you come to decide which ones you want.

Surgery

Surgery as an alternative to glasses or contact lenses is a controversial procedure. Perhaps I should say 'procedures' because several different types of surgery have been developed to combat short sight and even to correct long sight, although this latter is not as widely available.

Surgery of this type, called *refractive surgery*, is relatively new and basically involves changing the curve of the clear cornea which, with the help of the lens, bends light rays so they focus on the retina (see chapter 2). Short-sighted people have large eyes so the light is brought into focus in front of the retina (see Figure 3.5); they have too great a curvature in their cornea for the size of their eye, which results in distant objects looking blurred. Refractive surgery can be used to flatten the cornea by the required amount. Long-sighted people have too small a curvature in their corneas for the size of their relatively small eyes and as a result have difficulties with near vision. Surgically increasing the curve of the cornea is more difficult than flattening it but it can be done.

Pioneering work was done in the Soviet Union in the late 1970s, and in the early 1980s a technique was introduced called *radial keratotomy*, which is better known as RK. The technique involved making deep cuts round the edge of the cornea with a special scalpel and so flattening it out. The operation was not taken up immediately by eye doctors in the West because of a lack of information from the USSR at the time with regard to complications and the effectiveness of the procedure. Subsequently it has been shown to be effective. It is a common refractive surgical procedure used in the USA at the present time and it is sometimes used in Britain. However, for the unfortunate, the procedure does have some complications.

In Britain different types of operation are preferred by surgeons and one of these is *photorefractive keratoplasty* or PRK. In this operation, which is done under local anaesthetic, the surface epithelium is removed from the centre of the cornea and a furrow is cut out of the underlying stroma very precisely with a special type of laser (see chapter 1 for the structure of the cornea). This surgery is very much at the 'leading edge': the surgeon is in charge, but the laser is under the direct control of a computer which has been primed with all the information needed to make a furrow of the appropriate size to cause the required amount of flattening. PRK makes other forms of surgery, even keyhole surgery, seem very crude.

RK and PRK, no matter how sophisticated they may be, are surgical procedures and all surgical procedures may have complications and unpleasant side-effects. Fortunately severe side-effects are rare with both procedures, but they do happen: for example, sometimes with RK the cuts can be too deep and the correction is not what was hoped for. A side-effect of both procedures is that the eye is extremely painful when the anaesthetic wears off; the cornea is one of the most sensitive parts of the body, as you will know if you have had a poke in the eye – and this is far more than just a poke in the eye! A large number of patients suffer from glare after PRK, which is minor problem for most but for some people it can be severe. There is still considerable debate among eye professionals on the rights and wrongs of subjecting people with perfectly healthy eyes to a procedure which might risk that health, no matter how small that risk might be.

Refractive surgery is only available on the National Health for patients with specific eye illnesses. The short-sighted and the long-sighted who want the procedure as an alternative to glasses or contact lenses will have to pay. Most operations are undertaken by private clinics but they are also carried out in some NHS eye departments. Private clinics usually charge considerably less for refractive surgery than hospital eye departments, but the latter usually have a far longer period of follow-up after treatment. Usual practice is to operate on one eye at a time, doing the second when the first eye has recovered.

The question is often asked as to whether surgery is the way ahead for those with weak sight and whether contact lenses and glasses are things of the past. Basically it boils down to whether or not it works, and whether or not it is safe. Refractive surgery certainly works but it is not the miracle treatment for weak sight that is often claimed. Where there is a large correction, it will bring down the power of the lenses required, but glasses or contact lenses will still be needed. Even if the correction is perfect, some healing will occur in the cornea after surgery, which will counter the flattening for the short-sighted. In other words there is some regression with time; how much depends very much on the individual.

Such surgery has some risk so it is not entirely safe, but severe complications are fortunately rare in both RK and PRK. This, however, is no comfort for those who had a healthy eye to begin with, but sadly suffered such a complication. The surgery can be said to be as safe as any procedure that alters the eye, but with the important proviso that these operations have not been performed for long enough for us to be entirely confident that all the complications and side-effects are known. Refractive surgery is still rapidly evolving and, for example, a new laser-based procedure called *LASIC* has been introduced in Britain in the past couple of years. LASIC supporters are confident that it is superior to other operations and it does not seem to have the glare problem associated with PRK.

Cosmetic refractive operations are here to stay as there will always be some people who will take the slight risk and the post-operative discomfort to rid themselves of glasses or contact lenses. If you are considering refractive surgery, then take objective advice. In addition, one of the questions to ask the doctor who is going to do the procedure is 'Would you have it done yourself?' In my own hospital the specialist in PRK sports a very conventional pair of glasses!

A VISIT TO AN EYE DEPARTMENT

The clinics and departments

If you need to go to an eye department, the simplest way is with a letter from your GP (or in some regions from an optometrist). On the other hand, there are times when it is important to cut through the formalities and go directly to hospital, especially if you have had an injury or a sudden loss of vision or are in considerable discomfort. The two tracks lead into different parts of the hospital system.

The first, for people referred by GPs, leads to either a general eye clinic or a clinic called primary care (Figure 3.6). The object of this clinic is first of all to find out if there is anything wrong with the patient's eyes. If not, they will be given a clean bill of health. If there is something wrong, it will be treated there and then if possible; otherwise the patient is referred on to a specialist clinic for more specific evaluation and treatment.

Primary care, general and specialist clinics work on an appointment time basis, which means that delays in waiting time can occur, for example when patients require longer than the average allocated time or a doctor is off sick. (Patients who feel they have waited too long have recourse to the *Patient's Charter*.) The doctor may suspect what is wrong with the eye(s) but will undertake a thorough general inspection. Part of this inspection will involve equipment, some of which is described later in this chapter, and, if it is necessary to see into the back of the eye clearly, drops will be

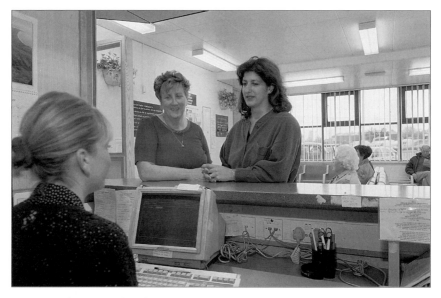

Figure 3.6 – The primary care reception at St Paul's Eye Unit, Liverpool.

required to dilate the pupil. It is best not to drive to the clinic, as if this happens, you will not be able to see clearly until the drops wear off.

Coming straight into an eye department without a GP referral leads to the accident and emergency department. This is a fast-track system designed not on an appointment or a first-come-first-served basis, but on a priority system whereby the most serious cases are seen first; those with less immediate eye problems have to wait. 'Less immediate' does not mean 'less important', but priority is given, for example, to those cases where delay could lead to further damage, babies with eye problems and so on.

All patients will be seen soon after they arrive by a special nurse called a *triage nurse* who decides who should be seen in what order. The triage system does mean that some people may have to wait a long time if there is a great deal of activity in accident and emergency (A and E), but all patients will be seen eventually. The problem will be treated there and then if it can be, so there may not be a need to come back; temporary or initial treatment will be undertaken with other patients who will then be required to come back at a later time, either to A and E or to an out-patients clinic, whichever is appropriate. Some emergency patients may need to be admitted to the eye ward, while still others will have eye problems that do not require immediate attention and will receive an out-patient appointment for further evaluation.

It is important to re-emphasize that attending an eye department does not mean that inevitably you will have to have an operation. By far the majority of patients who attend eye departments require drops or medication to control their eye problem and do not end up in the eye ward. Only one in ten patients attending an eye department ever comes to the operating theatre because of their eye problem. In recent years the trend in eye surgery has been away from operating under general anaesthesia, where the patient is put to sleep for the whole procedure. For this the patient has to come into hospital for a number of days. Where possible the operations are done under local anaesthetic and in these circumstances patients may only be in hospital for one day. They return home to recuperate with suitable support, only returning to the eye department for follow-up when required.

When patients realize that under local anaesthesia there is no pain and little discomfort, day case procedures are much preferred to staying in hospital for longer periods. Not all eye operations can be done under local anaesthesia and not all patients are suitable; this is a matter for discussion with the eye doctor if the need for an operation arises. Indeed some hospitals do not have day case facilities, but whether an operation is done under local or general anaesthesia, eye operations have an enviably high success rate.

The hardware

Ophthalmic and optometric equipment is becoming more and more complicated and sophisticated. Equipment for looking into the eye, for diagnosing disease, for monitoring eye conditions and for treatment can be large, alien and alarming for the patient. To the ophthalmologist and the optometrist the hardware comprises the familiar tools of their trade, but when they are busy they won't always have the time to explain it to unknowing patients in any detail. In this section I will mention some of the instruments and tests in common use.

Vision

Vision testing, similar to that in the optometrist's office, is an important part of an ophthalmic examination. Tests with the Snellen chart for distance vision will feature (see earlier and also chapter 2), and also near-sight testing with reading text will often be done.

Direct ophthalmoscope

The hand-held ophthalmoscope is the stock-in-trade instrument for the eye doctor and eye professional. It has a barrel with a flat top and the top contains a light and some small lenses. The doctor can use this in a number of ways, but will often hold it at a distance to see the front of the eye and how the pupil responds to light, or close to, to see into the back of the eye. This examination can be done with the patient sitting down.

Indirect ophthalmoscope

The indirect ophthalmoscope is a strange-looking contraption placed on the doctor's head and is used with the patient lying down. With the indirect and a special lens placed on the patient's eye, the specialist can see far more of the retina than is possible with a direct ophthalmoscope.

Slit lamp

Small tables with a chin support, a column of various bits and pieces and a set of binoculars are everywhere in an eye department clinic. These are *slit lamps* (Figure 3.2). The patient sits with his or her chin on the rest and the doctor or nurse uses the binoculars and a narrow slit beam of light to look in and around the patient's eye.

Tonometers

Tonometers are instruments for measuring eye pressure and you may have had experience in the optometrist's shop of one type which produces the puff of air (Figure 3.4). Eye doctors and their teams use a whole range of different types of eye pressure reading instruments. Some are hand-held and about the same size as the direct ophthalmoscope, while others have a box with them that produces a wavy line on paper or gives a digital read-out, but the most commonly used tonometer is a fitment that is attached to the slit lamp.

Each tonometer has a delicate probe which rests for a very short time in contact with the eye, except the air puff variety that optometrists use, which does not touch the eye. Such contact tonometers give more accurate eye pressure readings than the puff type and, personally, I find the sensation less disagreeable than the puff. The doctor puts a mild anaesthetic on your eye and also introduces a yellow-green dye called fluorescein which soon washes out.

Field analysis

The doctor may wish to check what can be seen out of 'the corner' of the eye, or the side vision (see chapter 2). The tests for side vision range from very simple doctor-to-patient evaluations, which give a rough idea of whether there is a defect, up to sophisticated machines called *perimeters* which can create a detailed map of side vision and pick up very early problems.

One simple test involves you sitting opposite the eye doctor, who will ask you to cover one eye and look with the other straight at his or her nose. The doctor stretches out an arm and asks you to say how many fingers are extended without moving your gaze away from the doctor's nose. This will be done in several arm positions for both eyes. The perimetry machines involve you looking at a point on a screen of some sort and being asked to identify spots of light which will appear in different positions. The most complex perimetry machines are computerized and are used on patients who have or are suspected of having glaucoma (see chapter 4).

Fluorescein angiography

Some eye complaints of the retina and its blood vessels can be diagnosed by injecting a yellow-green dye into the arm, letting it pass round to the eye and then taking a series of special photographs with a high-speed camera set up to look into the back of the eye. The yellow-green dye is the same *fluorescein* that is used for eye pressure testing (see earlier) and *angiography* just means taking photos of blood vessels. The doctor does not have the results of the test immediately; the film is developed and examined later for evidence of disease or abnormality. A side-effect is that the dye colours urine for a short time until it clears your system.

Lasers

Many sorts of *lasers* are used in ophthalmology, both for eye examination and for a range of treatments. Laser-based ophthalmoscopes are becoming more common in eye clinics for the examination of the retina and optic nerve, but they are much bigger and more complicated than more traditional ophthalmoscopes and not hand-held (Plate 9).

Other lasers are used in treatment of such conditions as diabetic eye disease (see chapter 4) and complications of cataract surgery. A laser can be used to bore a hole through the iris, which is done for certain forms of glaucoma. As mentioned earlier, a special laser is used for the PRK and LASIC procedures of refractive surgery.

Ultrasound

Most people will associate ultrasound machines with maternity clinics but, in the same way as they are used to examine the unborn baby, they are also used to look at the inner reaches of the eye, thus playing a part in diagnosis of eye complaints.

Electrical recordings

Electrical recordings help with diagnosis of heart problems and brain disorders, and can also be valuable in providing information on some eye complaints. The electrical activity of the eye can be measured, the activity of different components of the retina can be assessed and the activity in the visual pathway can be examined. Most of these tests involve the patient being hooked up to a variety of instruments by electrodes (which can be messy because of the contact grease, but they are not unpleasant), and a series of flashes or flickers are directed at the retina.

Eye help (first aid)

First aid for eyes, as with anywhere else in the body, needs training and there are many good training courses for those who are interested. On the other hand there are some simple things that are worth remembering which might stand the rest of us in good stead when faced with a minor eye problem.

Grit, a lash or something else can get into the eye and feel enormous, causing considerable discomfort. If it happens, then do not rub your eye: that is the worst thing to do because it might be a small jagged object that could lodge in your eye. The best thing is to blink furiously (see chapter 1) and allow the tears to wash the material clear – after all, that is your natural defence mechanism.

If someone has a foreign object in their eye and tears don't remove it, then you may need to look for the object. Wash your hands, get a clean linen handkerchief and place the person in good lighting conditions. With the thumb of one hand under the brow you can gently prevent the upper lid from closing, and with the thumb or first finger of the other hand pull down the skin under the lower lid to see as much of the eye as possible. Ask the person to look up, down and from side to side, and see if you can locate the object. If you find it, the corner of the clean hanky may be used to remove it, but if the object is embedded, you should take the person to the GP or to accident and emergency.

If the object is under the upper lid, you may need skilled help to dislodge it if tears alone are not working. One thing you can try is to grasp the upper lid gently between thumb and first finger, and then ask the person to look downwards. If you then very slowly bring the upper lid over the lower lid a few times, it might do the trick. In all cases you are only trying to remove materials which are not embedded in the coats of the eye. If they are stuck there, leave them alone and take the patient for professional help.

Black eyes result from bleeding into the tissues under the skin beneath and around the eyes. The discoloration is something you have to put up with, but the swelling, which can be very uncomfortable and can close the eye, can be reduced by crushed ice in a cloth. Crushed ice is much cheaper and more effective than the legendary steak!

Corrosives of any kind (such as acid or bleach) entering the eye can be a very serious matter and someone should call for an ambulance right away. However, while this is being done you can do the victim a great service by making sure they do not rub their eye and that plenty of tepid water is available to dilute the corrosive. Wash as much water as possible into the affected eye, being thorough but not rough; a gentle continuous stream of water from a tap may be more effective than trying to splash on water from a container.

VISION AND DRIVING

It is said by the College of Ophthalmologists that 95 per cent of the input from our senses to our brain that is needed for driving comes from our eyes. It is therefore not surprising that a visual check is an important part of the driving test. The basic vision requirement for the British driving test is 6/12 on the Snellen chart (see Figure 2.1, p. 27) using both eyes and appropriate glasses if necessary. The test itself of course does not use the Snellen chart; instead the candidate is requested to read a car number plate at a distance of slightly over 20 metres.

If a patient has failing vision there may come a time when the eye doctor considers that he or she is no longer fit to drive. The specialist will advise the person to notify the Driver and Vehicle Licensing Authority; this is not the doctor's job as it comes under a doctor's confidentiality to the patient. The specialist will write to the patient's GP informing of the eye problem and the lack of fitness to drive, but once again the GP can only advise the patient to give up driving, and only under extreme circumstances will inform the licensing authority.

It is exceptionally dangerous to keep on driving when you have a substantial visual defect as you are a menace both to yourself and to the public, but don't think that by going to the eye doctor you will automatically lose your driving licence. It is up to you to do the right thing if you are advised that your eyesight is no longer able to cope with the rigours of driving.

FACTS AND OLD WIVES' TALES

✧ Reading in poor light is not particularly bad for the eyes as many people are told. It will probably bring on a headache and is not something to be recommended, but it doesn't actually harm the eyes.

✧ Wearing glasses does not weaken the eyes or make them deteriorate in any way; all glasses do is compensate for what is lacking.

✧ Sitting too close to or watching the television in a very dark room may also bring on a headache, but again it is not harmful to the eyes.

✧ Some people wake up after a party and are missing a contact lens. If they are daily wear lenses then you shouldn't have gone to sleep with them still in! It is sometimes said that they can be lost 'behind the eye'. Contact lenses can't get round the back of the eye – the lens will be lying in your bed or on the floor, or lodged behind your upper lid.

✧ We rub our eyes far more than we are aware of, which is how pepper, onion, garlic, chilli and the rest can cause a nasty red eye. Wash with plenty of tepid water!

Chapter 4

Bad eye
The common eye diseases
and their treatments

This chapter will concentrate on the common eye diseases and their treatment. I have dealt with the various eye illnesses in alphabetical order and not in any order of perceived importance; after all, they are all important, especially to those who have them!

AGE-RELATED MACULAR DEGENERATION

Age-related macular degeneration, usually referred to as ARMD (or AMD), occurs in a number of forms, but the disease restricts itself to the macula, the delicate and vulnerable part of the retina of the eye that is most concerned with central vision (see chapters 1 and 2; also Plate 4). The macula is dominated by the cone type of photoreceptor and it is these macular photoreceptors which are gradually lost in ARMD – and with them goes central vision. Humans rely so heavily on central vision that ARMD is extremely visually disabling to those who suffer from the complaint.

Features and effects

ARMD is one of those eye conditions, like glaucoma and cataract, that arise in the elderly and develop usually in people aged 50 or more. Patients with ARMD often have a history of a gradual deterioration in vision over a period of several years. Also what normally would be seen as regular straight lines might to them appear wavy, for example, the side of a door, the top of a wall or the slats in a wooden fence. Reading can be a problem because the centre of the visual field (what the eye takes in when staring at something, see chapter 2) may be blank or blurred. People with macular degeneration don't go completely blind but they are visually handicapped and ultimately they have no central vision left at all. There can be a dark

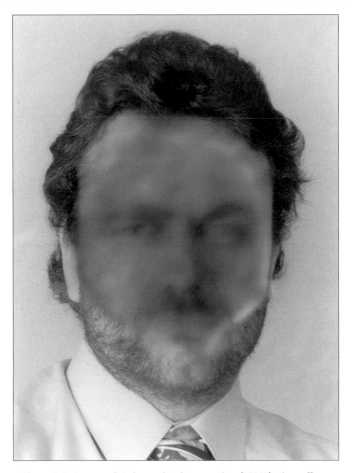

Figure 4.1 In age-related macular degeneration (ARMD), the sufferer
may have lost all central vision and see something like this, perhaps
with a slightly more foggy appearance to the central blank area.
(*Supplied by Mr Chopdar, Consultant Ophthalmologist to the Macular
Disease Society*)

and hazy area in the centre of the window of vision of an ARMD sufferer
(Figure 4.1). As the macula is concerned with fine detail, loss of its function
makes reading, writing and seeing small things extremely difficult. The
macula also dominates colour vision so, with loss of its function, colours
become much less bright, although their appreciation is not lost.

As people get older, material collects between the retinal pigment epithelial
cells and the choroidal blood supply. Remember that the epithelial cells
maintain the photoreceptors in good condition partly by supplying them
with what they need and partly by biting off the defunct outer segment
material that has become useless for vision (see chapter 1). This material

is partly digested by the cell, but remnants are extruded into the basement region called Bruch's membrane which separates the epithelium from the choroidal vessels. Over a lifetime the extruded material builds up and the membrane thickens; the thickening will happen in all of us but for some it will be the prelude to ARMD.

Types of ARMD

There are two main forms of ARMD called 'dry' and 'wet'. In ways that are not fully understood the thickening of Bruch's membrane is lumpy in some people and the lumps are prominent in the macular region. Not all people with these lumps will get ARMD, but a group of those who do also develop areas in the macula where the retinal pigment epithelium degenerates and dies in a slow withering process. These people have the dry ARMD and central vision slowly fades away; unfortunately the condition involves both eyes, although the degeneration can develop in them at different rates. Currently there is no medical or surgical treatment of dry ARMD that is known to be effective.

The second type, wet ARMD, develops more rapidly than the dry form and in this there is blood leakage from the choroidal vessels under the macula. This passes through the thickened Bruch's membrane and degenerate retinal pigment epithelium to distort and displace the macula. The blood leakage also encourages scar formation and these scars give rise to an alternative name for the advancing wet ARMD, i.e. *disciform degeneration*. If the scars and bleeding start at the outside edge of the macula and progress inward, effective treatment may be possible. A laser can be used to burn out the scar tissue and the areas of bleeding, and so halt the progress of the disease. For most patients, however, the scarring is dead centre on the macula and they cannot be treated without doing more harm than good. Lasers also have no beneficial effects on those people with the dry form of the disease.

Diagnosis and lack of treatment

If you are suspected of having ARMD you will need to see a specialist eye doctor. The specialist will check out your eyes generally, but will also dilate your pupil with drops. The specialist may think you should have fluorescein angiography, in which a yellow-green dye is injected into your arm and the doctor takes pictures very quickly of the back of the eye when the dye reaches it (see chapter 3). From these pictures the doctor can tell more about the state of the macula and whether or not it is the type of ARMD which can be treated.

The down side of ARMD is that the great majority of patients can't be treated, but the up side is that it is not a blinding disease. Vision will be poor, but ARMD sufferers are capable of going out and about as they will have all their side vision available. They should receive the support of a low vision therapist through attendance at low vision clinics. Help can be provided so that patients can adjust to get the best from their side vision. After all we spend all our visual lives being governed by central vision and it can be a tricky thing to suppress that dominance and let side vision take over. There are all sorts of low vision aids and devices available. Different people find different ones useful; it is a matter of trying them out.

Organizations such as the Macular Disease Society (address at the end of this book) are valuable, providing information, support and advice. One of my grandmothers had cataracts, but the other had ARMD, and let it get to her; she rarely left the house and was frustrated by her inability to read and write. She did not take to large print books or to tapes, and her ARMD made her very unhappy in the last years of her life. Perhaps if she had given low vision aids and support groups more of a chance, her quality of life would have been much better.

There are a number of conventional and alternative medical treatments that have become available and have been tried over the years, but none of them, with the exception of lasers, have proved to be effective. Personally I do not think that this depressing state of affairs is going to persist. Research continues at a pace such that new treatments like photodynamic therapy (PDT) are now being introduced into routine clinics in the UK and around the world. The PDT procedure treats the wet form of the disease by the use of a light-sensitive dye, which selectively gets to the abnormal vascular tissue, followed by special light exposure to the back of the eye. Under this combined assault, the troublesome vascular tissue shrivels up. However, the procedure prevents wet ARMD from getting worse only in a select group of patients. PDT is far from being a universal treatment for wet ARMD and needs frequent applications, but it is an improvement on laser burning because it causes far less retinal damage.

Much excitement has been caused by the fact that surgeons are now able to remove the abnormal vascular tissue from under the diseased macula, but unfortunately this has not brought visual improvement. The missing factor would seem to be the ability to replace, by transplantation, the degenerate retinal pigment epithelium. Techniques for retinal pigment epithelium transplantation are under investigation in many research centres around the world. Other surgeons have a different approach and that is to move the macula away from the diseased tissue and place it on normal support tissue. Surgery of this type is not easy and problems still have to be solved, so relocation surgery is not yet widely available although progress is being made.

Undoubtedly there is a genetic basis to ARMD but the family relationship is complex; suffice to say that there are some people who are more prone to the disease than others. ARMD became the eye disease of the twentieth century; it was not heard of before then. The reasons why the disease has come from obscurity to be the main cause of major visual disability in the western world is complex and a matter of considerable debate. One reason is that there are far more elderly people now and it is a disease of old age. Some eye doctors think that the modern western way of life contributes to the higher incidence of the disease, but if that is so then the key factors are not clear (see chapters 6 and 7). It should also be remembered that in the past ARMD may have been quite prevalent but merely not recognized as a disease in its own right by the eye doctors of that time.

CANCERS OF THE EYE

Various forms of cancer develop in the eyelids and in the orbital tissues which house the eye, but fortunately cancer within the eye is very rare (see chapter 5 on Sir Joshua Reynolds who suspected he had an eye cancer). Cancer cells from a site elsewhere in the body can settle in eye tissue and develop a lump, but there are only two cancers which develop first of all in the eye that are of any significance; one is *retinoblastoma* and the other is *ocular melanoma*. Neither form of cancer is particularly common.

Retinoblastoma

It is more than likely you will never have heard of retinoblastoma, which is an eye cancer of young children. This is not surprising because it occurs in about ten of every million children under five years of age. The cancer develops in the retina, probably arising from immature photoreceptor cells, and if it does occur it appears mostly in children under three years old.

The cancer has a whitish look about it and is picked up by the parents noticing a 'cat's eye' reflection of the normally black pupil. It can involve both eyes but usually only one. Often there is a family history but this need not always be so.

What was at one time a fatal disease is now successfully treated by *radiotherapy* or by special chemical agents, so that sufferers can expect in most instances to live to a ripe old age. Very small retinoblastomas can be treated by localized freezing. If the cancer is very big by the time the specialist sees it, then the eye may need to be removed, but the need for the loss of an eye is becoming less and less.

Melanoma

Skin melanomas have had considerable publicity in recent years because of their increased incidence, probably as a result of greater skin exposure to UV light for example through sunbathing and use of sun beds. It may not be so well known that a melanoma can also develop in the eye. The eye cancer is a separate entity in its own right; people with skin cancers don't necessarily get the eye cancer and vice versa.

Eye melanomas arise in the choroid (the blood supply under the retina), the ciliary body and rarely on the iris (see chapter 1 for the description of these structures). In all cases the cell of origin would seem to be a melanocyte, one of the pigmented cells found throughout these tissues, which are responsible for the colour of the iris. The choroidal melanomas are the most common of the three and usually appear in people over the age of 50. A choroidal melanoma grows beneath the retina and its increase in size causes retinal detachment. The loss of vision due to the detachment is the usual reason for the patient coming to the eye doctor. Remember though that retinal detachments are not uncommon, but this cancer is very rare.

If the melanoma is large, the eye is usually removed, but sometimes the surgeon will take out a small melanoma, leaving the eye intact and with some useful vision. In other circumstances, the cancer may be treated by special types of localized radiotherapy. Iris melanomas often do not grow much and are thought in the most part safe enough to leave, but if they change at all they are immediately removed by the surgeon, who takes out the piece of iris where the cancer is located (see *iridectomy* in the section on glaucoma). Treatment of ocular melanoma is a specialized business carried out by a few experts in the UK and most patients are referred to one of these by their eye doctor.

CATARACT

A *cataract* forms when the lens of the eye becomes cloudy and opaque; as a consequence light is gradually blocked off from the retina (see chapters 1 and 2). A cataract is not caused by a skin growing over the front of the eye as many people are still led to believe by their friends and relatives. Cataracts will develop as part of ageing, so the clouding will happen to all of us if we live long enough (Plate 10). About half of those over 65 will have some level of cataract development, but for many it will hardly be noticeable.

Hereditary and acquired cataracts

Cataracts are not always a result of ageing. Children may very rarely have cataracts which develop before or after they are born, and these are known as hereditary or developmental cataracts. Young diabetics can also develop cataracts (especially if their blood sugar control is poor) and additionally cataracts may form as a consequence of severe eye injuries or inflammation. Ultraviolet light can produce cataracts, so you must wear appropriate eye protection when using a sunbed. Infra-red light also can cloud the lens and a classic example occurs in glassblowers. If they stare too long and too often at the red, glowing, molten glass that they are shaping, then a cataract may be the consequence. Acquired cataracts of this type usually develop in the *lens cortex* away from the centre of the lens (see chapter 1).

Cataracts of ageing

The cataract of old age is called a *nuclear cataract* because the cloudiness develops right in the centre of the lens and slowly progresses outwards. As the cloudiness progresses, the centre of the lens hardens and becomes less capable of transmitting light to the retina. At first the cataract will not have a noticeable effect on vision; later on it will become a nuisance and if left too long it will be a major visual handicap. Older people first start to appreciate that they have the ageing or nuclear cataract on sunny days. When it is a bright day the pupil narrows down to restrict the light entering. However, when the pupil narrows, it centres on the very part of the lens which has became opaque.

The chemical changes which are associated with nuclear cataract formation are now well known and have been studied in great detail by scientists. Unfortunately what is not so well known is what factors are responsible for cataract formation in the first place. Also on the downside there is no conventional medication which either reverses the cataractous changes in the lens or even halts them. The treatment now, as it has been for thousands of years, is surgery, although there have been many advances since the couching and needling techniques originating in ancient India, which were still used by oculists in the eighteenth century (see chapter 3). All sorts of medical cures have been put forward, unfortunately too many by charlatans and the misinformed, but none has had the blessing of the medical fraternity or does any good at all.

Treatment

While there is presently no medical cure for cataract, cataract surgery is extremely effective for the vast majority of patients to the extent that it is one of the most successful operations available today. Procedures are continually evolving and they have come a long way since the treatment was the despised operation of barber-shop surgeons. The barber-surgeons pushed the lens to one side out of the visual pathway (see chapter 3). Later operations involved the removal of the lens, a procedure first pioneered by Jacques Daviel in the eighteenth century. The operation became progressively more sophisticated but there was an underlying problem. Without a lens the patient has +10D of long sight to cope with; in other words, the patient needs very thick focusing spectacles called cataract glasses to obtain a clear image. Contact lenses go part of the way to solving the problem but only part. The powerful spectacle lenses make everything look a little too big and there is edge distortion. Distance judgement is difficult, making steps a problem together with pouring tea and doing up laces.

Current operating technique has altered so that a plastic lens can be placed in the eye to replace the old cloudy lens, and the cataract glasses are then no longer needed. Recall that the lens is surrounded by a relatively thick clear membrane called the *lens capsule.* Modern procedures involve removing the bulk of the lens including all the cloudy material but leaving the capsule, which is like a bag, and into this the new plastic lens implant can be placed. The surgeon often uses an ultrasonic vibration machine to break up the lens into debris, which can then be removed by suction. Intraocular lenses do not remove the need for glasses, but the glasses required will not, in most cases, be the very thick ones of yesteryear.

Although cataract procedures have become progressively more complex, the disruption to the eye is less than it was because of a more delicate 'keyhole' surgical approach. As a result it is now common for patients to have their operations under local anaesthetic and to return home on the same day if they have people at home to look after them, although some may have to remain in hospital for a while (see also chapter 3). Some patients will require general anaesthetic and will also need to be in hospital for longer. This is something to discuss with the eye doctors beforehand.

All in all, cataract operations are highly successful and substantially reduce the impact of this type of visual impairment in the developed world. It is disastrous that on a world-wide scale so many people have untreated cataracts and cataract remains the major cause of blindness in the world today (see chapter 7).

DIABETIC EYE DISEASE

About 2 per cent of people will develop *diabetes* in their lifetime; it can begin in childhood but it also can have an onset later on in life, even appearing only in old age. Diabetics unfortunately cannot deal with sugar and carbohydrates in their diet because the cells in an organ called the pancreas no longer produce *insulin*. Insulin is an essential regulator of blood sugar levels and without it or appropriate medication the sugar levels in the blood will become dangerously high. Some diabetics need regular injections of insulin while others require tablets only; both need careful control of their diet. Diabetes is a serious illness, but it can be controlled to the extent that the sufferer has a normal quality of life and is hardly aware of the disease. As with any serious illness, however, there are complications which can occur and among these are eye problems.

Who gets eye problems?

The answer to this question is that the development of diabetic eye problems relates to the length of time that the person has had diabetes: the longer they have been a diabetic, the more chance they have of experiencing changes in their eyes. It is sad but true that 80 per cent of diabetic patients who have had their disease for 20 years or more will have eye changes. The changes may not be so severe as to create an obvious visual problem, but they are there and a check-up can reveal the tell-tale signs. The trick is to make sure that diabetics have an eyesight test frequently (once a year) and let it be known that they are diabetic; an eye test is free for anyone with diabetes and it is something the optometrist needs to know (see chapter 3). Also a GP may be involved with an eye hospital or diabetic early screening programme for visual loss, and anyone who has had diabetes for five years or more will want to be on such a programme (Figure 4.2).

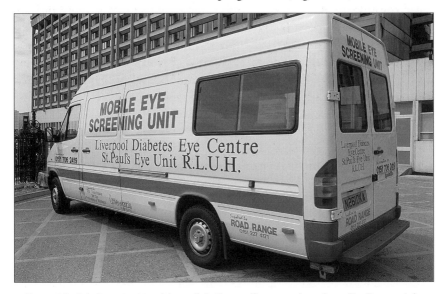

Figure 4.2 It is important to pick up diabetic eye disease early and monitor it accurately. St Paul's Eye Unit, Liverpool, for example, has a specially equipped ambulance which liaises with GP practices.

There are factors other than the duration of diabetes that are also important, such as the control of blood sugar levels; if this is poor then eye problems will develop more rapidly. The better diabetes is looked after, the more slowly eye problems will develop. Recent studies have shown that good control can reduce the risk of developing changes in the retina by half. If the diabetic patient has high blood pressure and this is not brought down to reasonable levels, then this is another risk factor for eye problems. Smoking is bad news, as is high alcohol intake. Diabetic women during pregnancy are at a heightened risk of some eye changes taking place. Eye problems can develop in both eyes, but one eye may be more advanced than the other. What are the eye changes that diabetics face?

Diabetic cataract

Young people with diabetes can develop a type of cataract exclusive to diabetics. Older diabetics develop age-related cataract (see 'nuclear cataracts of ageing' in the previous section), but more rapidly than their non-diabetic counterparts. Both types of cataract can be treated by surgery when required.

Diabetic (background) retinopathy

The most serious changes involve the retina and its blood vessels (see chapter 1). The first alterations can be seen by the eye doctor or diabetologist looking at the back of the eye, but they do not immediately effect vision. The small blood vessels in the retina develop weaknesses in their walls and bulge out. These vessels leak and cause local swelling; the leaking fluid can solidify to produce deposits in the retinal tissues. Bleeding from the leaking vessels will begin to be noted during check-ups, as will areas of tissue where the retinal nerve fibres have died. Eye doctors call these areas of dead neuronal tissue *cotton wool spots* as this is how they appear on examination. With progress of time the changes become more pronounced so that the bleeding and nerve death start to cause deterioration in vision.

Maculopathy

There is so much spare capacity in the retina as a whole that a great deal of damage can be done before it is appreciated as decreased vision. The one place where this is not the case is at the macula. Once the macula is involved in diabetic eye disease (*maculopathy*), the visual consequences of bleeding around it, deposits in it and macular swelling are partial or total loss of central vision.

Proliferative diabetic retinopathy

The proliferative part of the disease has the most severe visual effects. Proliferation is just another name for growth, and the things that grow at this stage of diabetic eye disease are new, thin blood vessels. The new blood vessels are formed at the surface of the retina and then grow into the vitreous humour (see chapter 1). The vessels are weak and bleed easily; bleeding into the vitreous humour will in itself cloud vision. In addition scar tissue is formed on the surface of the retina; the scars contract and detach the retina. The bleeding and the retinal detachment combine to produce a sudden decrease in vision; if left untreated there can be a total loss of vision in one or both eyes.

Severe cases of advanced diabetic eye disease can result in vascular scars forming on tissues away from the retina, for example, the iris and the aqueous outflow system. The vascular scar tissue can block the drainage of aqueous humour (see chapters 1 and 2), which leads to a severe form of glaucoma, *neovascular glaucoma* (see the section on glaucoma in this chapter). The glaucoma may be severe to the extent that the eye, already blind, becomes so painful that it has to be surgically removed to provide comfort.

Treatment

The earlier diabetic eye disease is picked up, the better the outcome is likely to be. The very earliest changes do not require any treatment but as the disease progresses and vessels start to leak it is necessary to undertake laser therapy (see chapter 3). This will be done as part of a special outpatient clinic. The patient will have two sets of drops administered, one to widen the pupil while the other is an anaesthetic. The laser is fitted to a slit lamp and its light is used to seal the leaking blood vessels. A special contact lens is fitted to the eye to be treated and the laser gives out a series of bright flashes.

If the diabetic eye disease is advanced to the stage when there are newly forming blood vessels, the laser will be used to get rid of them also. Removing the vessels can be rather uncomfortable, so often a painkilling tablet is given before treatment, but if this is not enough a supplementary injection can make all the difference. Often several sessions with the laser are required to allow the eye doctor to treat every possible point of concern on the retina. After a laser session it will take a day or so for vision to return to normal in the treated eye.

If the disease process has reached advanced scar formation with retinal detachment and bleeding into the vitreous humour, something other than laser therapy is needed. What may be required in this situation is complex eye surgery, although this is not appropriate for all patients with advanced eye disease. Microsurgical procedures have been developed whereby the vitreous humour, clouded with blood, can be extracted and the retinal scar tissue removed. After this any points of bleeding can be treated, either at the time of surgery or later. It must be pointed out that such procedures are not always successful and visual improvement may not be possible. Diabetic eye disease accounts for more than a thousand blind registrations per year in Britain and remains a major cause of blindness in the developed world.

GLAUCOMA

Glaucoma is not one illness but a family of conditions that have features in common, namely: an elevated pressure within the eye; loss of visual field; and cupping of the head of the optic nerve where it enters the eye. The most common form of glaucoma in Britain, western Europe and the USA is called *primary open angle glaucoma* (POAG) or chronic simple glaucoma. There is another form of the disease called *closed angle glaucoma* (CAG), which is common in Asian countries including Japan. Many forms of glaucoma exist as a complication of another disease process and these are called 'secondary'. In addition there is a form of glaucoma in babies and children known as *congenital glaucoma.*

Primary open angle glaucoma (POAG)

This form of glaucoma has a slow onset and is particularly common in the elderly. Normal eye pressure (*intraocular pressure*) is around 16mm Hg higher than the outside (atmospheric pressure), but this slowly creeps up through the 20s into the 30s in those with this form of glaucoma. Eye pressure is created by the clear liquid inside the eye called aqueous humour which is continually secreted into the posterior chamber of the eye, passes forward into the front (anterior) chamber and from there passes through a biological drain back into the blood (see chapters 1 and 2). In open angle glaucoma the drainage tissue gets blocked by a mechanism that is still not understood and this leads to a high pressure within the eye (Plate 11A and B).

When the pressure increases it can damage the delicate fibres which take information from the retina back to the brain through the optic nerve. They are particularly vulnerable where the nerve enters the eye and, under the twin assaults of too much eye pressure and poor local blood flow, this nerve head collapses to form a cup, killing the delicate fibres. The more fibres that die, the more vision is compromised. POAG affects side vision first of all, and only much later does the patient start to lose central vision. The slow onset and tunnel vision mean that sufferers are often not aware that they have a problem. Most glaucoma is picked up first by the optometrist on routine visits to check glasses (see chapter 3). It is therefore very important to go to an optometrist who does a pressure test when you are over 40 years of age, especially if you know of someone in your family with glaucoma because the disease does run in families. Eye tests are free for those in this age group who have relatives with glaucoma because they are at slightly increased risk.

Primary open angle glaucoma is a complicated disease which still baffles us in many ways. There are people who have the glaucomatous loss of vision and the damage to their optic nerve head, but have no high eye pressure. These patients have low or *normal tension glaucoma* and often slip through the net of routine pressure checks. It is likely, but not proved, that their eye disease relates more to vascular problems at the back of the eye rather than pressure problems as such. To make things even more difficult there are many people with higher than normal eye pressure who fortunately never seem to suffer visual loss. They are termed *ocular hypertensives* and show that glaucoma cannot be diagnosed simply on the basis of having a higher than normal eye pressure. High eye pressure is just a risk factor.

Nonetheless there are many people with glaucoma who remain undiagnosed and lose far too much vision before they are ever seen by an eye doctor. Hence the importance of having an eye pressure test regularly if you are over 40.

When someone has POAG, they are prescribed drugs to lower eye pressure and for most people this is extremely effective. Unfortunately the vision they have lost is lost for ever, but further visual loss can be prevented. A whole battery of medical treatments are available; some reduce the rate of fluid production within the eye and others help to open up the drainage system so that the eye fluid can clear more effectively. If drugs fail, then laser treatment of the drain is an alternative, but a surgical procedure, called a trabeculectomy, to create a bypass route for the fluid to exit the eye is the option of choice. Trabeculectomy is now a highly successful procedure with relatively few complications, although as with any surgical technique it is avoided unless there is no alternative.

Closed angle glaucoma (CAG)

CAG also results from blocked fluid drainage from the eye, but here the cause is the iris being pushed forward by the build-up of fluid behind it. The fluid responsible for eye pressure is produced by the ciliary processes and reaches the front chamber of the eye through the pupil (see chapters 1 and 2). The space between the lens of the eye and the iris bordering the pupil is small, but in some people it is particularly so. These are the people at risk from CAG because the opening can close altogether and create a pupil block. The fluid builds up behind the iris and the delicate tissue is pushed forward by the weight. The iris billows out like a parachute opening and eventually blocks the main drain for exit of fluid from the eye, situated in the recess of the front chamber called the chamber angle (Plate 11B), hence the name 'closed angle glaucoma'. The result is that eye pressure increases so that the visual system is threatened.

Eye pressure can reach very high levels very quickly and this causes the acute form of the disease. The acute attack can be very frightening because the sufferer often becomes disorientated and nauseous. Open angle glaucoma is painless but the acute closed angle attack may be painful and is definitely uncomfortable. The important thing is to get to a hospital eye department as quickly as possible. There the sufferer will be given pills or eye drops to drastically reduce the production of fluid into the posterior chamber and so reverse the tendency for the iris to block the chamber angle. Medication is only a temporary solution until surgery can be undertaken.

The surgery, an *iridectomy*, involves taking out a small segment of iris tissue to make a bypass for fluid to pass directly from the posterior to the anterior chamber without needing to go through the pupil. The procedure can be done either by conventional surgery or using a laser, which avoids the need to enter the eye. If the equilibrium is re-established quickly the iris falls back into its correct position and the pupil block is reversed. The operation may not work if the lowering of pressure and the surgery are not soon enough after the attack has started. Inflammation within the eye leads eventually to adhesions forming between the iris and the drainage tissue. In this case, after iridectomy the iris will not be able to fall back from the chamber angle and open up the drainage pathways. Treatment thereafter becomes far more difficult.

With some people the angle closure is partial and progressive, the drainage pathway slowly becoming blocked as the iris steadily 'zips up' the anterior chamber angle around its 360 degrees. It is this form of closed angle glaucoma which is common in many parts of Asia.

SECONDARY GLAUCOMAS

There are a large number of different types of secondary glaucoma but fortunately they are not common. Essentially they fall into two groups: those where material blocks the drain – like tea leaves in a sink – and those which can produce angle closure with the iris. In the first group a severe form of glaucoma results from excessive release of iris melanin which clogs up the drain, causing pigmentary glaucoma. Blood cell debris, lens substance and inflammatory cells can all produce their own forms of secondary glaucoma, and there are many others. In the second group, the iris can billow up into the drainage angle following injury or disease (see James Joyce in chapter 5). Some diabetics with eye disease can develop a form of glaucoma called *neovascular glaucoma* (see the section on diabetic eye disease). Here scar tissue and new blood vessels grow on the surface of the

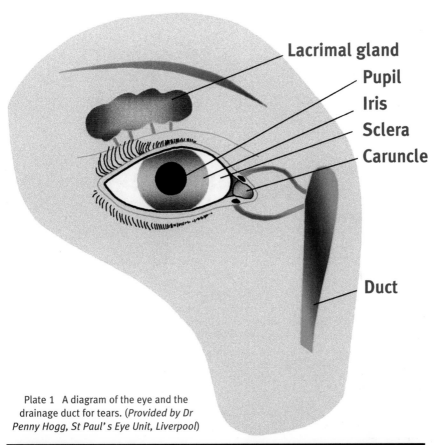

Lacrimal gland

Pupil

Iris

Sclera

Caruncle

Duct

Plate 1   A diagram of the eye and the
drainage duct for tears. (*Provided by Dr
Penny Hogg, St Paul's Eye Unit, Liverpool*)

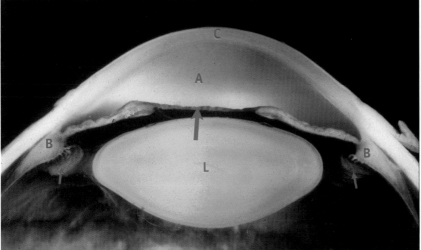

Plate 2   The front of the eye in section showing the cornea (C), the anterior chamber (A),
the pupil (arrow), ciliary body (B), ciliary processes (small arrows) and the lens (L).

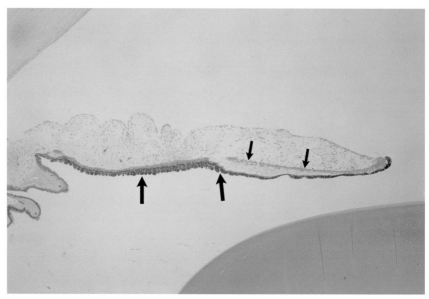

Plate 3 A stained section through the iris. The sphincter muscle (small arrows) and the pigmented epithelium (large arrows) are marked. The epithelium really consists of two layers but looks like one at this magnification.

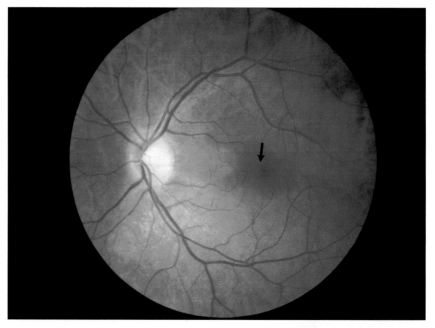

Plate 4 Looking into the eye and through the pupil with an ophthalmoscope, the red of the choroid can be seen through the clear retina. The optic nerve where it enters the eye is seen as a white disc with blood vessels running from it, and the macula can be identified as a spot on the retina (arrow).

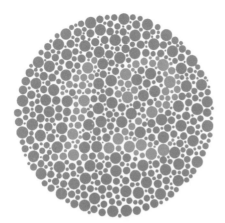

Plate 5 The first picture from the Ishihara colour vision test. The orange 12 can be seen by both people with normal colour vision and those with colour deficiencies, but later pictures in the series distinguish between the two.

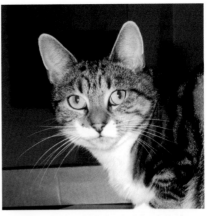

Plate 7 The cat has good night vision but tends to be dazzled in daylight. The eyes have oval pupils which can narrow down more effectively than the round ones of human beings.

Plate 6 (*right*) Circles and ovals within a circle look like nothing, except perhaps breakfast eggs and sausages? Arrange them differently within the circle and the very powerful face image appears.

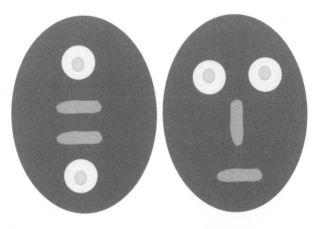

Plate 8 (*below*) Some extracts from the iridologist's chart.

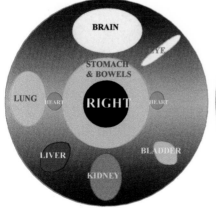

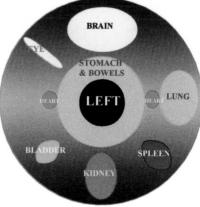

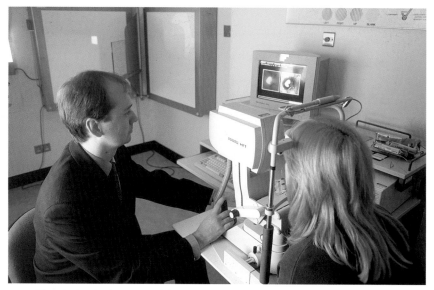

Plate 9   An eye doctor examining a patient with a scanning laser ophthalmoscope.

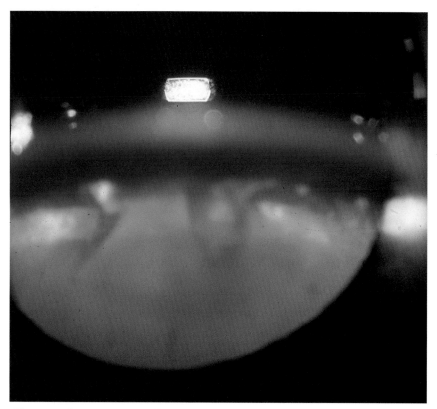

Plate 10   A dense cataract seen by using a slit lamp. In a normal eye the lens would be clear.

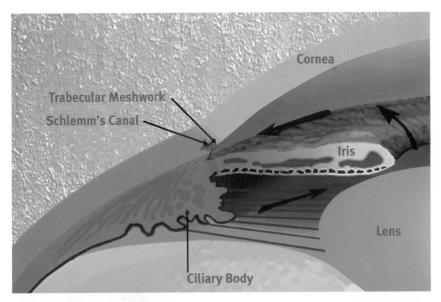

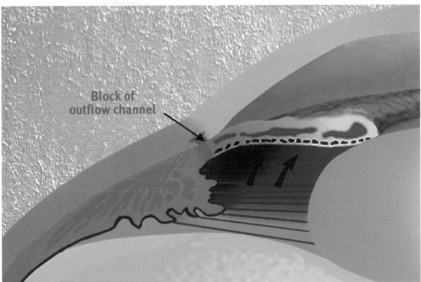

Plate 11 (A) Eye pressure is higher than normal in primary open angle glaucoma (POAG); it is caused by poor flow of aqueous humour through the outflow system. (B) In closed angle glaucoma (CAG) the eye pressure is much higher than normal and this is caused by the iris blocking the outflow system. (*Provided by Pharmacia & Upjohn, UK*)

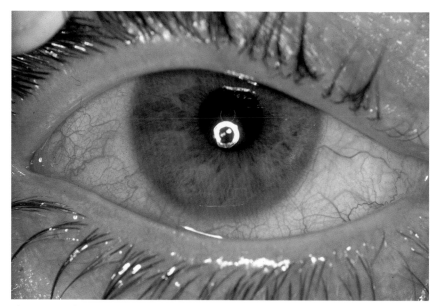

Plate 12 A red eye. The inflamed conjunctiva in conjunctivitis has prominent blood vessels and the eye is watery.

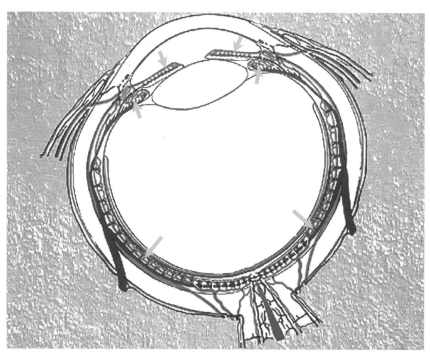

Plate 13 The blood vessels of the choroid (arrows) together with those of the ciliary body and the iris (small arrows) collectively make up the uvea.
(*Provided by Pharmacia & Upjohn, UK*)

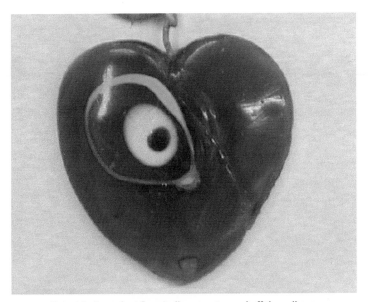

Plate 14   A pendant from India, worn to ward off the evil eye.

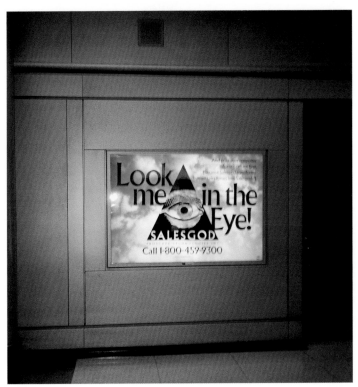

Plate 15   Advertising is not just words; it is intended to have an impact on our feelings, often through powerful images. What more powerful image is there than the eye itself?

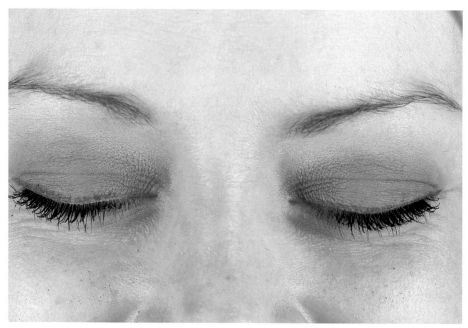

Plate 16   Even beautiful eyes can take an extra bit of help with eye make-up.

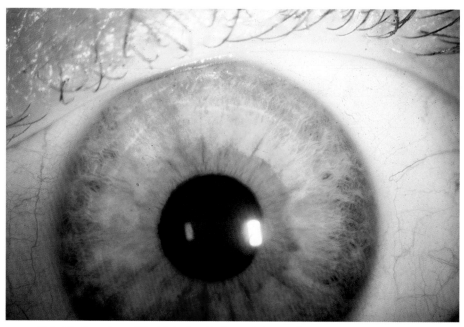

Plate 17   The colour of the iris in the elderly can fade, usually remaining relatively bright
around the pupil, but fading more toward the edges.

iris and this new tissue contracts causing the iris to scrunch up. As it scrunches up, the drain is impeded and glaucoma results.

Congenital glaucoma

Congenital glaucoma is rare and unpleasant. A very small number of babies are born with their drainage system underdeveloped or malformed. The more severe the defect in the drain, the earlier in life the glaucoma arises, so it can appear in the newborn or late on in childhood. Babies with glaucoma can have enlarged protruding eyes because the high eye pressure distends the pliable coat of the young eye. Treatment of congenital glaucoma usually involves surgery of various types to assist with aqueous drainage.

ONCHOCERCIASIS (RIVER BLINDNESS)

A dreadful name for a dreadful illness which thankfully does not occur in Britain, although it is rampant in West Africa and other parts of the world such as Central America. *Onchocerciasis* is the technical name but it is better known in the tropics as *river blindness*. In the villages along the many rivers of West Africa large numbers of people will be blind or visually handicapped as a result of this disease. As well as causing considerable hardship to its victims, river blindness exacts a high price from the villagers who have to support friends and family members who are no longer capable of work or of looking after themselves. The villagers who have the burden of having to support their blind and partially sighted relatives and neighbours are often hardly capable of maintaining much of a standard of living for themselves.

The worm and the fly

The disease is caused by a small worm called a *filarial worm* which is passed from the infected to the healthy by a biting *blackfly* species, for example in Africa it is the buffalo gnat. The blackfly lives in the vegetation near to water and the maggots of these flies thrive in water close to fast-running rivers where they remain until they pupate into flies. The blackfly therefore is very restricted in its range because of the association with fast-running streams, which is just as well because otherwise river blindness would be even more of a problem than it in fact is.

The blackfly 'injects' immature worms into the skin of a human it bites. There they grow into adults and become surrounded by a tough cyst which can be seen as a lump on the infected person. The worms live for many years and produce vast numbers of larvae called *microfilariae*. The larvae migrate through the skin and some are taken up by other blackflies that bite the infected person. The larvae become immature worms in the flies and are passed on to other people in turn. The mobile larvae in the skin cause rashes and itching; skin colour may be lost particularly on the legs, and in severe cases of infection the irritation leads to the skin becoming scaly, thickened or wasted. The consequences of heavy infection are not restricted to the skin, and the eye problems give rise to the common name of the disease, river blindness.

Eye problems

The larvae may reach the eye, particularly in heavily infected people, and invade many of the eye tissues including the cornea, iris, choroid, retina and optic nerve (see chapter 1). It seems that the damage is not caused so much by the living mobile larvae, but when they die they produce local inflammation and tissue destruction. These little disruptive 'time bombs' cause particular devastation to the delicate tissues of the eye. Visual impairment and blindness occur through several mechanisms. The cornea can cloud over and become scarred, the infected retina and choroid degenerate, and the optic nerve head wither – any one of these would produce blindness in its own right.

Treatment

In some areas all the population is infected with the worms and of these, about 10 per cent will be blind or partly blind. Most drugs that are used to kill the worm have been of little value until recently when a drug called ivermectin was introduced. Ivermectin stops the adult worms producing larvae and, as that is the key to the problem, it has been a considerable success so far. Another advantage of the drug is that it only needs to be taken once a year. Through the combination of ivermectin to attack the worm and carefully planned eradication programmes to reduce the incidence of blackflies, it is hoped that river blindness will not be the problem in the future that it is at present.

RED EYE

Red eye, of course, does not have a single cause but is a symptom of many problems, some trivial, some extremely nasty. A red eye is the most common eye problem that is seen by GPs and it is also the main reason why people come to an eye unit's accident and emergency department at hospital (Plate 12). Here I will only cover a few of the many causes of red eye; others may be mentioned elsewhere in the book, for example a serious sight-threatening cause of red eye is an acute attack of closed angle glaucoma.

Each of us can probably remember looking into a mirror and seeing a horrible red eye reflected back at us by the glass. Everywhere you go people will comment on how sore it looks: sometimes they are quite right, and at other times it looks far worse than it really is. With red eye we are dealing with a whole range of things which produce an 'itis'; superficially they look the same, but their origins differ as do their most effective treatments. Remember the 'itis' at the end of a medical term denotes an inflammation of whatever tissue is named at the beginning of the term, for example, an inflammation of the conjunctival membrane of the eyeball (see chapter 1) is *conjunctivitis*.

Infectious conjunctivitis

In this condition, one or both eyes have a very red conjunctiva due to inflammation which makes the vessels in this thin membrane swell and then leak. The eyes feel gritty, with an itchy or burning sensation, they water all the time, there may be discharge and in some cases dark glasses are needed to protect against bright lights. These are typical features of both *infectious* and *allergic conjunctivitis*. An infectious conjunctivitis is produced either by bacteria or by a virus.

Bacterial infection is usually indicated by a yellowish discharge in the inside corner of the eye and a crust in the eyelashes which sticks the eyelids together in the morning. Bacterial conjunctivitis usually clears up of its own accord in a week or two at the most, but a doctor will give drops to help limit the bugs, chloramphenicol being a favourite. However, what is a minor problem for most people can be a little more problematic for those with contact lenses. Chloramphenicol is mild and simply prevents the bacteria growing, so contact lens users may need something stronger, for example gentamicin, which actively kills the bugs. Lenses should not be worn until the infection has cleared completely, but they should be taken to any appointment with an eye doctor as they may prove useful if the infective organisms need to be further identified. Bacterial conjunctivitis is unpleasant but not sight-threatening – with the exception of the chlamydial form that leads to trachoma (see later).

Sufferers of viral conjunctivitis have a watery discharge, often very copious, rather than the sticky discharge that is usually associated with bacterial infection. Grittiness may well be very evident and patients tend to be extremely light-sensitive. Viral conjunctivitis may be associated with flu-like symptoms or a sore throat, but as often as not there is nothing at all. The eye doctor looks under the lower lid of the patient for little lumps in the red membrane (part of the conjunctiva). The lumps are a feature of viral infection.

Viral conjunctivitis cannot be treated as such, much like that other 'incurable' virus, the common cold. Instead its symptoms are relieved as much as possible, with painkillers if needed, and cold compresses bring some comfort. It usually takes a little longer to clear up than the bacterial form. Viral conjunctivitis is highly infectious so disposable hankies should be used, while pillows, towels and such like need to be kept separate and washed frequently. Eye doctors themselves contract more than their fair share of this infection through patient contact. Viral, like bacterial, conjunctivitis is unpleasant rather than sight-threatening.

Allergic conjunctivitis

There are roughly equal numbers of patients who come to eye departments with the allergic and the infective forms of conjunctivitis. As stated earlier, the symptoms are similar for both. An important set of patients within the allergic group are the contact lens wearers who develop an allergy due to exposure to their contact lens solution (see chapter 3). Changing the type of solution may solve the problem but, if not, it may mean that contact lenses will be inappropriate thereafter.

Dog hairs and pollen are often the cause of red eye, but unfortunately for the vast bulk of allergic conjunctivitis sufferers, the root cause of their inflammation will remain unknown. People who are prone to allergic conjunctivitis tend to suffer from hay fever or asthma. For many, the allergic conjunctivitis will be a periodic or, in the case of pollen allergy, a seasonal inconvenience requiring occasional anti-inflammatory eye drops. On the other hand there are particularly sensitive people who tend to have extremely severe and persistent bouts of conjunctivitis; they need a great deal of additional out-patient care.

Keratitis

Just to make things a little complicated, an inflammation of the cornea is not 'cornitis' but *keratitis* (for some perverse reason best left to the medical profession).

Corneal inflammation can arise from a number of causes such as injury and the presence of foreign bodies (see later), severe dry eye due to an absence of tears, infection and ulcer formation. The infections can be the same as those in the conjunctiva and are treated in much the same way. The cornea keeps bacteria at bay as long as it is healthy and not injured, but with an injury to the surface epithelium the opportunist bugs can gain entry into the tissue and, if they are allowed to thrive, a white area develops in the clear cornea and a painful ulcer can occur.

Viruses produce keratitis and also corneal ulcers called *dendritic ulcers*. During the examination the eye doctor uses a dye to show whether there is an ulcer and how big it is. The virus lives in the nerves and can damage them so that corneal sensitivity is reduced. This is not good news because the cornea needs to be sensitive as part of its defence against the outside world. If either viral or bacterial keratitis is not brought under control with drops, scarring can occur and with scar formation comes an invasion of blood vessels from the surrounding tissues. Both the scarring and blood vessel invasion conspire together to make the cornea opaque (an extreme version of this is described later in the section on the disease *trachoma*) and so result in loss of vision. A corneal graft operation to substitute a clear cornea from a donor may be the only solution. Corneal grafting has the distinction of being the most successful transplant operation of all, but the eye doctor would work hard to avoid such a drastic measure.

There are other 'nasties' apart from bacteria and viruses which can invade the cornea and produce keratitis. If fungal spores get into the cornea they can produce a nasty reaction and may even start growing. Fungus can't gain entry into the cornea in the normal course of events, but an eye injury due to a stick or the thorn of a rose sometimes carries spores into the wound. There is an organism called *acanthamoeba* which lives in water but is becoming a menace to contact lens wearers. It seems to like contact lenses and their cases, and it is not killed by the weaker disinfectant solutions. Fortunately it is not very common, but cases of amoebic infection are becoming more frequent each year. The amoeba likes to live in still water and thrives in the cold water tank in the loft and also in the hard-water crust on taps. *Never* clean your contact lenses or lens case with tap water; this fellow and his bacterial friends can do a great deal of damage to your eyes!

Iritis

Iritis is an inflammation of the iris and it gives a redness to the surrounding tissues, thus producing a red eye; the redness is usually most obvious where the clear cornea and white sclera merge together (see chapter 1). The eyes do not have a discharge but may well be watery. Patients are often extremely sensitive to bright light, they have an ache in their eye and there may be some blurring of their vision.

Iritis sufferers are unfortunately subject to periodic bouts of inflammation and will have a very small pupil, particularly if they have had previous attacks.

Episcleritis and scleritis

The sclera is the white of the eye and it can look red in conjunctivitis because of the swelling of the blood vessels there. However, the sclera can become inflamed in its own right. *Episcleritis* involves only the most superficial part of the sclera and inflammation here is uncomfortable but a minor problem. *Scleritis*, involving the whole structure, is more serious and it is persistent. It seems mostly to be associated with joint and connective tissue diseases of the rest of the body such as *rheumatoid arthritis*.

Injury

A sharp injury can lead to a foreign object damaging the cornea, being stuck in the cornea or even penetrating beyond the cornea into the inner reaches of the eye. All of these situations result in the defences of the eye being breached and the possibility of corneal infection by any of the bugs mentioned previously. A whole host of objects in the home, garden, workplace, etc. conspire to harm the eye. Small children's fingernails become dangerous weapons to the unwary parent. Pen and pencil injuries are common in both children and adults. Safety goggles worn in the workplace are forgotten by the DIY expert at home. The garden seems a less tranquil place when you consider the number of injuries from trees and thorns that are seen at accident and emergency. There are still too many people at work who remove their safety equipment for a moment and get hot sparks, metal fragments or similar objects in their eyes.

Blunt injuries, resulting from anything from fists to balls, distort the eye and cause internal bleeding, plus a very red eye. The internal bleeding frequently looks worse than it really is and this blood often clears quickly through the outflow system (see chapter 1). If such injuries are severe, tears in the retina and even retinal detachment can develop. Being hit by tennis balls and fists can lead to sore eyes which look worse than they really are, because much of the impact is absorbed by the brow and the cheek. Smaller objects, such as corks from fizzy wine bottles, golf balls and squash balls, can often do much more damage because they avoid the eye's outer defences.

Chemical injuries caused by acids and strong alkalis can cause horrendous damage to the eye. These are not just a danger to the eye in a chemical factory or other such premises; strong bleach, oven cleaners and battery acid from cars all too often claim victims among the unwary.

RETINAL DETACHMENT

The retina is a fragile structure, and perhaps the most delicate part of it is the bank of photoreceptors lined up and held secure by the retinal pigment epithelium (see Figure 1.7). It is here that a retinal detachment will start, as a separation of the retinal photoreceptors from the supporting pigment epithelium. The retinal pigment epithelium, the underlying vascular choroid and the fibrous wall of the eye (the sclera) are robust. All three help to protect the delicate retina, as does the jelly-like vitreous humour which fills the cavity and clings firmly to the retina's inner surface. The firm support provided by the outer walls of the eye and the vitreous jelly acting like a shock absorber combine to provide the retina with the best of protection. In all but an unfortunate few the retina stays firmly in place for a lifetime.

The pigment epithelium holds on tenaciously to the retinal photoreceptors, but the region where they meet is inevitably a place of weakness simply because of the differing strengths and rigidities of the tissues involved. As we get older, the strong connection between the vitreous jelly and the retina is reduced in areas for reasons eye doctors still do not really understand, and this means that the shock absorber is less effective than it once was. Older people are more susceptible to detachment than the young, but it is a matter of degree. Short-sighted people with larger than normal eyes are also more prone to detachment.

The precursor to detachment is the formation of a hole in the retina that can come through injury (see chapter 5 on Frank Bruno) or because the individual is born with a particular tendency to form retinal holes. Areas that are particularly prone to detachment are those where a hole or holes have developed in the delicate retinal tissue. This is because these holes bring an additional weakness to the structure by allowing fluid to accumulate where the retinal pigment epithelium and photoreceptor layer meet. The association between the pigment epithelium and the photoreceptors can be likened to a zip-fastener, which is strong only as long as it is completely intact; once it is breached it is especially weak. Thus a retinal hole is like a tooth missing from a zip: gradually and relentlessly the whole thing starts to unthread.

I'm told that people experiencing retinal detachment most often feel that a shadow comes over what is seen from the affected eye; also black spots called *floaters* can become very obvious, bobbing across their vision. We all have floaters and see them against a light surface when we are tired; to have a few is a normal sign of ageing, but many appearing suddenly are not, so anyone experiencing this should go to their doctor, if only to eliminate the prospect of a detachment.

Treatment

As with many of the eye conditions discussed in this and other chapters, it is important that a doctor sees and treats a retinal detachment as quickly as possible. For the retina to function it needs its close contact with the retinal pigment epithelium and the nutrition provided by the vascular choroid; this is particularly true for the photoreceptors. Without that contact the well-being of the retina as a whole and the survival of the photoreceptors, so crucial to vision, are in jeopardy. A detachment has to be treated as soon as possible, if good vision is to be retained once the retina is back in position. If the central retina and macular region are involved in the detachment, then visual loss from the initial detachment will be dramatic and, unfortunately, full recovery is unlikely. It is for this reason that the most urgent cases of detachment are those where only the edge vision is involved (an indication that the macula is still attached and hopefully will remain so).

There is no medical treatment for detachment, although a patient may well be given medicine to reduce any inflammation that may have arisen during the detachment. The treatment for retinal detachment is surgical. There are a whole host of procedures available, but the underlying essential step is to identify where the retinal holes are located and then to close them. Without closure of the holes, more fluid can seep into the retina, with the consequence that successful and permanent reattachment of the retina is not possible.

Prominent among the surgical procedures to treat holes and breaks in the retina is a freezing procedure. The eye doctor uses a probe which is placed on the outer wall of the eye at the appropriate site. This produces localized 'frostbite' in the tissues around the hole; over time this then becomes a permanently sealed scar. Alternatively a laser may be used to 'spot weld' around the hole; its beam is directed via lenses to the appropriate spot inside the eye. Mostly the external freezing and the laser process are done under local anaesthetic.

The retina may need to be encouraged to make good contact with the wall of the eye. This can be achieved by the surgeon fitting a silicone band and sponges on the wall of the eye close to the detachment. If the eye doctor is not satisfied that the hole has been secured and the detachment is on its way back into position, it is likely that a special type of gas will need to be injected into the eye so that a bubble forms over the detachment and retinal break, effectively sealing the break. In order to keep the gas bubble situated over the break, the patient might have to stay in a restricted position for a while. In some circumstances an internal operation will be required because the eye doctor needs to tackle the torn area from inside the eye and also remove the vitreous humour which can become troublesome.

In the past there were awful stories about patients having to stay in bed for week after week with minimal movement so that their detachment had the best chance of repair. This sort of torture did occur, but now most retinal detachment patients who have had the full operation are a little uncomfortable for a couple of days and need to stay in hospital for that period. Thereafter they are up and about again with no ill effects. Often detachment patients are mobile the day after their surgery, which is rather different from the case in the past (see chapter 5 on Gordon Brown).

Complex surgery

The treatments mentioned in the previous section are effective at reattaching the retina for around nine of every ten people with detachments. For the 10 per cent that are less successful, it is because scar tissue develops inside the eye, preventing the retina from reattaching, or making the detachments even bigger and in some instances tearing the retina. It is ironic that one of the cells most involved in the scarring process is the retinal pigment epithelium, which starts to increase (not like a cancer), moves into the vitreous humour and helps make the scars. If there was ever a case of friend turned to foe, this is it.

Surgical treatment for these complicated cases is long and involved. However, retinal reattachment can be achieved with some visual improvement in a number of cases. Much more can now be done than was possible only a few years ago. These patients, along with those who have severe ocular injury or end-stage diabetic eye disease, are among the most challenging that the ocular surgeon faces. They tend to be treated by eye doctors who specialize in *vitreoretinal surgery* and are at the front line of new skills and surgical technology.

Other detachments

Detachments due to retinal holes have taken up most of this section because they are the most common, but there are others. As mentioned in the section on ocular melanoma, these growths and other cancers beneath the retina can develop and push the retina away from its normal attachments. In situations where there is severe inflammation within the eye, particularly when it involves the choroid, fluid can leak from the choroid into the retina and break the connection between the photoreceptors and the retinal pigment epithelium to produce a detachment.

Damage to the choroid, through blunt injury for example, can produce bleeding which results in a local detachment. More severe penetrating injuries to the eye can produce internal scars which contract and detach the retina. As noted previously, in the end stages of diabetic eye disease massive scars can rip the retina away and produce an extensive detachment. The detachments produced by scarring require extensive and very specialized eye surgery if any sight in these eyes is to be saved.

RETINITIS PIGMENTOSA

The retinal diseases that belong to the *retinitis pigmentosa* (RP) group are mostly, but not always, inherited and are not particularly common. The different variants of the disease are often associated with different types of inheritance through families. There is one type in which all the children of an RP parent have the disease but it develops only slowly. Another type finds only a few offspring affected, but for the few the disease is severe and blindness is rapid.

The name of this disease is misleading: the loss of vision does not result from any inflammation of the retina (retinitis) but is brought about through a degeneration which involves the photoreceptors and then the retinal pigment epithelium. It is a tragic family of diseases resulting in the death of the photoreceptors; the rods are more vulnerable and the cones survive longer, but eventually all are lost in both eyes.

The complex and intimate relationship between the photoreceptors and the retinal pigment epithelial cells, which 'nursemaid' the rods and cones (see chapter 1), breaks down in RP and the related degenerative diseases. The orderly stacks of discs involved in the photochemistry of vision become disrupted and the retinal pigment epithelium is no longer able to keep its rods and cones clean, tidy, safe and well. Understanding the molecular and genetic basis of the disease was one of the successes of the 1990s. Numerous genetic variants have been identified in affected European families, but in the USA, RP is much more genetically conservative. To explain the contrast it has been suggested that RP has arisen in Europe as a consequence of several different genetic events. These diverse events have all resulted in the same thing – a progressive failure of the photoreceptor to function properly. The preponderance of one genetic form in the USA has led to the speculation that much of the RP in that country arose from one immigrant family: there is some evidence that one of the original Founding Fathers on the *Mayflower* had or carried RP.

Unavailability of treatment

The molecular and genetic investigations have furthered our understanding of why people get RP and who will get the disease. They have not as yet brought a cure or a treatment to halt the inexorable progress towards blindness. It is hoped that the new knowledge will open the door to the development of the first generation of RP treatments, but whether these will be medical, genetic or surgical remains unknown. Numerous claims regarding effective treatments have been made in the past, but all have been either premature or bogus.

The people

The onset of RP occurs early in life, but not so early that the sufferers do not appreciate the full benefits of good vision that is then cruelly taken away. Their sight is not snatched away, but disappears slowly; these young people have to face the relentless loss of sight, which starts, in its most common form, as poor vision in dim light (the early loss of rods), progresses to tunnel vision (rods predominate in side vision, see chapter 2) and ends with little or no vision at all (the last of the cones are lost). This usually occurs in the childhood years and early adulthood. It might seem easy to give in to this malicious handicap, but in my experience quite the opposite occurs. RP sufferers do not tend to let their visual loss stand in their way. I have an RP friend with whom I worked for many years who is a gifted computer programmer; another is a communications lecturer at university. If you have RP or have a friend who has it, do contact the Retinitis Pigmentosa Society (see end of book for address).

SQUINT (STRABISMUS)

The technical term for *squint* is *strabismus,* but there are other less flattering terms heard in day-to-day use, for example, 'cast' or 'cross eyed'. Some controversies about squint and its management (conventional and otherwise) have been mentioned in chapter 3, but here, I will cover it in a little more detail. In every pre-school group of 40 children, 3 can be predicted to have some level of squint. It is a major problem that keeps the children's clinics of hospital eye departments at full stretch.

What is squint?

Think of the eyes of a young baby: they move all over the place but rarely together. After the baby reaches six months of age, control kicks in and the eyes start working together in unison, the control getting better as time goes by. For some children the control does not seem to work very well (*latent squint*) or it does not work at all (*manifest squint*). Squint can take several forms, for example, when the stronger eye is fixed on some object, the squinting eye can turn outwards (Figure 4.3A) (*divergent squint*) or the squinting eye can turn inwards (Figure 4.3B) (*convergent squint*); turning up or down are also options. By far the more common childhood squint is the convergent, which is three or four times more frequent than the divergent.

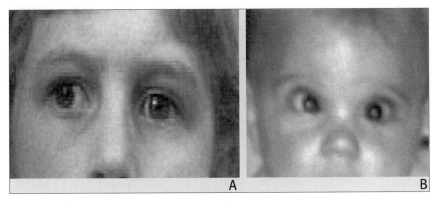

Figure 4.3 Squinting eyes: (A) a divergent squint where the eye turns outwards and (B) a convergent squint where the eye turns inwards. (*Provided by Gail Stephenson, Head of Orthoptic Department, University of Liverpool*)

Binocular vision requires both eyes to work together to allow the slightly different images from both eyes to be fused together in the brain. The problem with the squinting eye is that it gives confusing information to the brain, resulting in a fuzzy or double image. The brain soon learns to suppress the image from the squinting eye and take information only from the stronger eye. This is not a good outcome. Remember that in the young child, central vision and macular function are just becoming properly established (see chapter 2) and will not develop properly in the squinting eye unless it is made to line up with the stronger eye. If suppression is allowed to continue, the loss of vision in the squinting eye will eventually become permanent – a condition known as amblyopia (or *lazy eye*).

Treatment

The basis of treatment is to get the eyes in alignment, reverse the suppression and obtain the best vision possible from the weak eye. Working with the eye doctor on this are the hospital optometrist and particularly the orthoptist (see chapter 3). The sooner treatment is started the better (under three years of age is recommended by my paediatric colleagues): if the squint remains for a long period, the loss of sight may well became permanent. As a rule of thumb, children whose squint is not treated until they are over six years old do much less well than the younger ones (they have a lazy eye).

The visual problems are corrected with glasses and for several weeks the child has the good eye covered (a patch or tape on the spectacle lens is favoured) so that the weak eye has to do all the work. Children, who may already experience bullying or name-calling because of their squint, may receive even worse treatment at this stage. Older children dislike patching intensely, but the very young ones may not tolerate it at all. As an alternative, drops can be used in the good eye to dilate the pupil as wide as possible so that its image is not as sharp as usual, and this will make the weak eye do more work. However, I'm told that this is a poor substitute for patching.

Some children, usually the older ones with latent squint, do very well as a result of eye exercises arranged and taught by the orthoptist. These exercises need to be done regularly if they are to do any good. If a squint is obvious, however, the eyes may only get back into alignment after an operation performed by a paediatric specialist eye doctor. The doctor will operate on the muscles of the weak eye or even the muscles of both eyes if need be. In this type of squint there is nothing wrong with these muscles, they are not sick or damaged in any way, but altering them can bring the eyes into alignment. An immediate and worthwhile cosmetic benefit comes as a result of squint operations, even if visual improvement in the weak eye is not always what had been hoped for.

Paralytic squint

The bulk of childhood squint is the result of a problem between eye and brain; there is nothing wrong with the extraocular eye muscles, which move the eyes up and down and side to side (see chapter 1). There is, however, another type of squint called *paralytic squint* where one or several muscles are damaged so they cannot work very well. This type of squint can occur in adults as well as children. The damage to the muscles can be the result of hereditary problems, injury or disease. For example, sometimes squint can develop in a baby delivered using forceps after a long labour, whereas in an adult, eye muscle damage can result from a head injury. Fever and illnesses in childhood which involve high temperature can damage eye muscles and result in a squint. Meningitis, multiple sclerosis and myasthenia gravis are a few among a long list of illnesses which can bring on paralytic squint.

TRACHOMA

Trachoma is the third most common cause of blindness in the world today and is close behind glaucoma in second place (see chapter 7). It occurs as a result of an eye infection caused by a micro-organism called *Chlamydia*. The organism and its associated eye disease are common throughout the developing world, but are most rampant in the warm, dry desert regions of the Middle East and North Africa. In these areas, whole communities can have trachoma but in very varying degrees of severity. Children are subject to multiple bouts of infection; no sooner do they recover from one round of chlamydial infection than they contract another. Some individuals experience a very mild infection while in others it is particularly severe; why this should be is unknown.

How do you get it?

The disease is associated with poverty and poor living conditions where good personal hygiene is hard to maintain. Trachoma is frequently spread, for example, by sharing towels and also it is thought to be passed on by flies going from the eyes of one person to another. All in all, there are thought to be over 500 million people with the disease and somewhere between 1 and 2 per cent go blind, while an even higher percentage have a serious visual handicap. It is young children who have the most active form of the disease and are so prone to infection and reinfection. In adults, it appears that women are far more prone than males to later infection and also to the onset of blindness, probably because they are the ones looking after the children, who have the most active disease.

The illness

When it enters the eye, the micro-organism produces an inflammation of the conjunctiva (conjunctivitis, see earlier) and after time the conjunctival membrane thickens. Small lumps form under the eyelid and there is some superficial scarring on the clear cornea. Eventually the infection will disappear and most of the scarring will heal. Unfortunately any immunity the sufferer has developed does not seem to last very long and reinfection can set in. It is the continuous cycle of infection and reinfection that has the most serious visual consequences.

The corneal scars become more extensive with reinfection. In addition, in a dry, dusty climate, the grit and wind can be unbearable irritants, making the swelling and soreness considerably worse. Other secondary eye infections, both bacterial and viral (see the section on red eye), can set in and have a more devastating effect than they would in healthy eyes. The scarring starts to cloud the cornea and also blood vessels grow down on to the cornea to compound the problem. Repeated trachomal infection causes the lids to tighten and bend in, and as a result the lashes start to rub the unhealthy cornea. The rubbing causes further pain and also produces ulcers. In the end the cornea is completely opaque and the patient is blind.

Treatment

The chlamydial micro-organisms live inside the cells of the eye and thus are difficult to treat, but nonetheless they are killed by some antibiotics, including tetracycline and erythromycin used in the form of eye drops. In advanced cases, where the lids and eyelashes are folding in on the eye and causing damage to the cornea, surgery on the lids may be needed or, at the very least, the offending lashes need to be removed. Where possible superficial opaque scar membranes are surgically detached. The problem is that often, particularly in remote regions, there is insufficient medical support to provide any of the necessary services (see also chapter 7).

Eyes west

Although trachoma is rare in developed countries, it is by no means absent and the micro-organism is becoming more common. Although trachoma has been a problem in Britain in the past (see chapter 5 on William Wordsworth), today chlamydia is associated not so much with eye problems as with sexually transmitted disease. There is an increasing incidence of people with genital chlamydial infections and this can act as a reservoir for eye contamination. For example, newborn babies can develop eye problems if their mothers have genital chlamydia.

UVEITIS

The *uvea* is the main bed of blood vessels in the eye, consisting of the choroid (beneath the retina), the blood supply to the ciliary body and the blood supply to the iris stroma (see chapter 1 and Plate 13). If the choroid becomes inflamed the result is *choroiditis*, while ciliary body inflammation is *cyclitis* (iritis has been mentioned before, in the section on red eye); if more than one of the three are involved, the result is *uveitis*. In practice uveitis is a common end point for a vast array of different entities and conditions, only a couple of which I will mention here.

Choroiditis

Choroiditis can be patchy and also involve the retina, leaving behind it ugly scars. Often the cause is unknown but one form of choroiditis is produced by a worm called *Toxocara*. You may have heard of this because it is often in the news; it is the worm that is passed on, usually to children, by contact with dogs' faeces. Not surprisingly, given the state of parks and gardens, most of us become infected with the eggs of the worm and build up resistance to them. Children with a lack of immunity are vulnerable to infection, but fortunately it is only a very few who get the worm in their eyes. Even then there is only minor damage as long as the scars are away from the central retina and the macula in particular. If, however, the scarring does involve the macula, the visual loss can be severe.

I love dogs but have a low opinion of many dog owners and their selfish disregard for other people. Of course, the risk of eye disease from fouling of public places is extremely low, but there should not really be any risk at all. Puppies particularly can have very high worm burdens and all dogs should be regularly wormed with a tablet from the vet to reduce the hazard.

Sympathetic ophthalmitis

It is a cruel twist of fate that a severe injury to one eye can lead to visual loss or even blindness in the other undamaged eye (see chapter 5 on James Thurber). If the injury causes extensive damage to the uveal tissues, the body can react via its immune system to eye components that it mistakenly thinks are foreign organisms. Once the immune system is primed in this way, which can take anything from a month to a year, it makes no distinction between the bad eye and the good eye, and attacks each with equal ferocity. Repeated attacks from the body's defence system can lead to total loss of vision in the once good eye.

Today *sympathetic ophthalmitis* is very uncommon because of prompt treatment and suppression of the initial inflammation by steroids and the like. It is, however, still advised that badly damaged eyes with no vision at all should be removed within a fortnight of the injury, certainly less than a month later, to remove any possibility of a sympathetic reaction in the other eye.

Vitamin A deficiency

Vitamin A is one of the essential vitamins mentioned with respect to night blindness in chapter 2. It has an important role in the formation of visual pigment for the rod photoreceptors of the retina, the receptors responsible for vision in dim light. Some people with a mild deficiency in vitamin A can have poor vision at night which is helped by taking additional vitamin A in the diet. In this section I will, however, discuss profound vitamin A deficiency, which is an altogether different matter and is suffered by too many of the underfed children in the developing World.

What goes wrong in the eye?

Vitamin A is not just essential for the visual process; it is also needed for the proper functioning of surface epithelial cells, particularly in their production of mucus. Mucus seems like nasty stuff, particularly when you have a cold, but it has an important role in the normal functioning of tissues and nowhere is it more important than in the eye. A thin layer of mucus produced by the conjunctiva helps to keep the tear film in place on the surface of the cornea (see chapter 1). Children who are malnourished and have a major shortage of vitamin A in whatever diet they have are prone to epithelial problems, and the epithelium of the conjunctiva and the cornea is the most vulnerable area. The sufferers have a dry eye, not because they have no tears but because the tear fluid has no mucus to stick to. The dryness is only one symptom and the main problem is the development of severe corneal ulcers. The cornea seems to melt away and then scar over, leading to blindness.

Prevention

Around 250 million children in the world suffer from severe nutritional problems which could lead to the blindness associated with vitamin A deficiency (see chapter 7). The vitamin is found in abundance in eggs and liver, and it can be formed in the body from a plant material called carotene, which is of course associated with carrots, but other foodstuffs such as tomatoes and greens are a rich source. Obviously children who are poor and malnourished will not have ready access to eggs and liver, but surprisingly in areas of northern India and other places where vitamin A deficiency is a real problem, green leafy plants abound but are rarely used as a food source. Nutritional education could make some inroads into this distressing condition.

FACTS AND OLD WIVES' TALES

✧ I have often heard people saying that their cataract has 'grown back' after surgery. This is not the case: once the lens is removed it cannot grow back, but in some people fibrous tissue can cloud up behind the implanted plastic lens some time after cataract surgery. The surgeon then undertakes a simple procedure, using a laser to remove the fibrous film on the plastic lens.

✧ The idea for using plastic lenses inside the eye came from the Second World War. During the Battle of Britain, perspex from shattered plane canopies entered the eyes of some pilots during dog fights. Eye doctors were surprised to find that the eye tolerated the plastic rather well and it was on the basis of this experience that they first thought of plastic lens implants.

✧ It is a scary fact that diabetics are ten times more likely to go blind than non-diabetics. If you have diabetes, make sure your eyes are checked regularly.

✧ You don't have to have high eye pressure to develop glaucoma and not everyone with high eye pressure has glaucoma.

✧ Contact lens wearers develop red eye as an allergic reaction not to their lenses but to their washing solution. All users should take care to clean the solution off before inserting their lenses in their eyes.

✧ Straining the eyes will not give anyone a retinal detachment.

✧ If a child has a squint, they will not grow out of it: squints do not go away of their own accord.

Chapter 5

Who am eye?
Famous people who have had
eye problems

In chapter 7 I will address the world problem of blindness and visual handicap, but in such an exercise there is a tendency to forget that poor vision is a challenge that an individual has to face in his or her own way – hopefully with all the support that a caring society can give. Loss of a sense is a very personal tragedy. I believe it was Sir John Wilson of the World Health Organization who said, 'People do not go blind by the million. They go blind individually, each in his own predicament.' In this chapter I want to concentrate on individuals, famous people from the past and present, who have had to cope with the handicap of blindness, visual impairment or even just a minor ocular imperfection, and its consequent effect on their lives.

RELIGION

St Lucy

In the Middle Ages in Europe medical treatment was at a low ebb: little could be done for most ailments, but there was one source of healing which is still used today, namely the power of faith and the Church. Someone with an eye problem in the Middle Ages might be treated by a travelling oculist, who would probably be a dangerous quack (see chapter 3). Alternatively they could pray to a healing saint or, even better, go on pilgrimage to a church or shrine that had holy relics of such a saint. There are several healing saints who are associated with blindness and failing vision, but probably the best known is St Lucy.

St Lucy is the patron saint of the blind. She is said to have lived in the fourth century AD and to have been born into a Christian family in Syracuse. Being a Christian at this time was dangerous and her troubles began when she was engaged to a man she did not like. The fiancé wanted Lucy to give up Christ but she stubbornly refused, and in a rage he denounced Lucy to the authorities. She was tortured but she held steady. At one point she asked the prefect in control of Syracuse, who was her main oppressor, what he most admired about her. He said without hesitation that her eyes were her best feature. It is said that she promptly plucked them out and sent them to him.

Pope Leo X

One of the most powerful families in Renaissance Italy, the Medicis were the driving force behind the growth and prominence of the city state of Florence. They were described as a highly intelligent but not particularly healthy family. In addition it seems likely that many in the family were short-sighted, some extremely so. Lorenzo the Magnificent (1449–92), one of the best known of the Medici, was often described as having poor or weak sight and is known to have had prominent eyes. It is generally the case that short-sighted people have larger than normal eyes (see chapter 3). Lorenzo's second son Giovanni became Pope Leo X (1513–21) and he was definitely short-sighted because the –12D concave lens that he used to see distance is still kept in a museum in Florence. In a famous painting of Leo by Raphael he is shown clearly holding his lens.

Short-sightedness or myopia has through the years been considered a weakness. However, it was no such weakness to the Medici family, who gained vast power, wealth and influence, exemplified by one of the family members becoming pope and another being the powerful Queen of France (Catherine de Medici). It has been said that if the Medici family had had normal sight they would have become soldiers and generals. Saved from that, they were able to concentrate on politics and making money, and you could therefore say that their poor sight was the key to their great success.

MILITARY

Blindness and visual impairment are a risk to the military. I include two famous examples, and one less famous.

King Harold

King Harold did not have to cope with a life blighted by blindness or visual impairment, but he is a very powerful historical symbol of an extreme eye problem in a military context. It was King Harold who died as the result of an arrow in his eye at a crucial moment in English history. (Although as a schoolboy I always confused him with King Alfred – the one who allegedly burnt the cakes.)

Harold came from a very powerful Anglo-Saxon family with some claim to the throne of England. When Edward the Confessor died in 1066 without an obvious heir, Harold had himself crowned king. His claim was disputed by his brother Tostig, and by the King of Norway, the Duke of Normandy and a whole host of others. Tostig and the King of Norway landed in the north of England and Harold had a famous victory at Stamford Bridge during which both his enemies were killed. No sooner was this battle over than Harold heard that the Duke of Normandy, William, had landed near Hastings.

Harold's tired army was sorely depleted through battle casualties and desertions by the time it reached the south of the country, but Harold was determined to fight William as soon as possible. It was William who started the battle by an attack on the disorganized English army perched on the high ground, but the Battle of Hastings was not to be decided on one attack; it was to be a long drawn-out affair. The English shield wall was faced by the triple threat of Norman men-at-arms, cavalry and archers. The English were more than a match for the foot soldiers and could even hold the cavalry (William had three horses killed under him), but the archers were a real problem.

The Norman archers poured arrows into the shield wall and, late on in the battle, Harold was hit in the eye by one of them. He pulled out the arrow and tried to continue to fight, but it was a serious wound and soon all the king could do was hold on to his shield. Finally the Normans broke through the English shield wall which had held so firm all day, Harold was killed and the battle was lost. The image of Harold with that arrow in his eye has persisted throughout history, but it must be said that evidence for it happening is not that strong. The best evidence is from the famous Bayeux Tapestry in Normandy, which depicts the course of the battle and shows Harold with an arrow in his eye.

If we assume that this tale is true, was the arrow the deciding factor in the battle as we are often told? It is difficult to say. At that stage the English were extremely hard pressed and very depleted in numbers, so they might have crumbled anyway. However, it also must be said that the Normans had been repulsed all day long and they were also ready to crack. Harold's eye injury coming at such a crucial time would have had a bad effect on his weaker troops, who then began to desert the battle in droves. An injury to the leader was a disaster for morale. Much earlier in the battle, it had been rumoured that William had been killed and it took all of William's effort, riding backwards and forwards without his helmet on, to convince his soldiers he was alive and that they should not panic.

Harold's best troops were his own guards or housecarls. Their job was either to get the king away safely from the battlefield or to die defending him (or, if he was dead, his body). The housecarls were the cream of the English fighting men, as they had proved in this battle and at Stamford Bridge, but they were wiped out to a man. The eye injury was a double blow: it caused panic and desertion in the English army at a key point in the battle, but it also meant that the honour-bound housecarls could not get their badly injured king away and therefore were also doomed. The Battle of Hastings was a close-run thing but, once over, it left the Normans as the new masters of England as no English force was now strong enough to stand against them. Norman influence had a profound effect on the development of Britain, so an eye injury may have been a turning point in its history.

King John of Bohemia

In the years up to and beyond 1346 the English were the scourge of France: small, well-disciplined armies harried the French countryside in the name of their king, Edward III, who claimed the throne of France for himself. It was in 1346 that Edward landed in France with a modest army of 12,000 which included his son, the Black Prince. He was eventually confronted near the village of Crécy by a huge French army, well in excess of 30,000 strong, dominated by knights on horse and the elite of the French nobility.

The English army was of a different composition. There were some knights on horseback, there were many seasoned men-at-arms, but the core of the army was the archers, who used the longbow as their main weapon. The Black Prince, Edward Prince of Wales, was given command of the right side of the English army and this was where much of the action was to be focused. First of all, crossbowmen were sent forward by the French to engage the English, but they were obliterated by the far more effective English archery. Next came the French cavalry charge headed by, among others, blind King John of Bohemia. Despite their armour and their undoubted bravery, the cavalry were no match for the lethal showers of arrows that rained down on them. The many cavalry charges were shattered and the demoralized and disorganized French army was routed. Among the mounds of dead was King John.

I first heard of the Battle of Crécy, the triumph of the Black Prince and the death of King John, during school history classes and it fascinated me in a morbid sort of way. I tried to imagine how awful it must have been to be blind and have, despite the affliction, to lead an army of mounted knights into battle against a determined enemy. King John was in charge of the second wave of cavalry in the French army. He was dressed in full armour and mounted on a large war horse, as were all those around and behind him. John would hear the clanking of all the metal, the neighing and snorting of the horses, and would have been quite disorientated were it not for those retainers there to guide him.

Soon after the start of the battle the crossbowmen, who were sent in first, and the front line of cavalry were in trouble. John didn't hesitate and committed his men to a charge. There was a roar as the charge began; perhaps he shouted a few war cries himself to keep his spirits high. During the charge he would be aware of the pounding hooves behind him and the vibrations in the ground, like a mini-earthquake; was he also aware of the increasing excitement in the knights around him?

They went through the disheartened, retreating French soldiers and Genoese crossbowmen; did John think they were the enemy? Very soon after, the real enemy would strike, causing confusion and disorder, shouting, crashing men, frightened bewildered horses as shower after shower of lethal arrows hit them time and time again. Could blind John have had any real idea of what was happening to them all? What was he doing in such a conflict? After all, win or lose, his chances of survival couldn't have been good.

Medieval society was governed by rules of duty which made knights and even kings, irrespective of disability, fighting men required by feudal oath to defend land and country. Simply, some of John's troops were committed to fight for the King of France and if they had to fight so should he. He was clearly a brave man who in success would have been a hero but in crushing defeat became a byline in history. The irony was that, at Crécy, sighted or otherwise, none of the French army had any control over what went on that day. The French had never faced this type of warfare before but they would face the same horror of lethal archery at future battles with the English, ending with Agincourt nearly 70 years in the future. Blind King John had a very distinctive crest of ostrich feathers which the Black Prince adopted and it has been the prominent part of the badge of the Prince of Wales ever since.

Admiral Lord Nelson

If you had to name a British naval hero, Nelson (1758–1805) (Figure 5.1) would probably be rivalled only by Drake at the top of most lists. He was a prominent, and then later the dominant, figure in Napoleonic sea battles, which included Cape St Vincent (1797), the Nile (1798), Copenhagen (1801) and the greatest sea battle of them all, Trafalgar (1805). The deck of an eighteenth-century fighting ship in action was not a place where injuries were easily avoided. Nelson had more than his fair share of these, which included losing his right arm, but his first serious injury, the loss of the sight in his right eye, was not gained aboard ship at all.

In 1794, Nelson was captain of a ship of the line, called the *Agamemnon*,

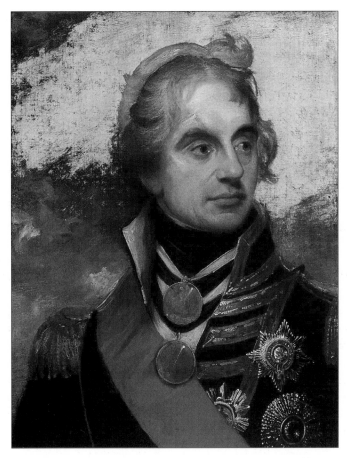

Figure 5.1 Admiral Lord Nelson in 1800. The right eye was his damaged eye. (*By courtesy of the National Portrait Gallery, London*)

which was based in the Mediterranean. He was sent with troops to Corsica, to siege towns and fortifications there. At one town called Calvi, Nelson was supervising the installation of guns on shore when a cannon ball from the town struck his battery. He was hit in the face and upper body with stones, sand and wooden splinters. One of the splinters cut through his right eyebrow, through the lid, and unfortunately penetrated his eye. He was in great pain but the surgeon, who removed the splinter and dressed the wound, thought that his sight would be saved. Despite such a severe injury, Nelson was back on duty the following day. Four days later he reported that his wound was much better, but the vision in the damaged eye had deteriorated from being reasonable at the outset to only allowing him to distinguish light.

Perception of light was the best Nelson would ever get from his right eye from this time on and the eye was to be sore for months. At the end of this period, the pupil was extremely dilated to the extent that an observer could hardly see his blue iris in that eye, and the pupil remained dilated, being no longer reactive to light. In addition the pupil was no longer round but irregular. The splinter on entering the eye may or may not have lodged in his iris, and no doubt more damage was done by the surgeon removing the splinter in field hospital conditions.

Either at the time of the initial wound or as a consequence of splinter removal, the ocular fluid (aqueous humour, see chapter 1) would have been lost out of the injury site. It may be most likely, because initially Nelson's sight seemed to be reasonable and then deteriorated, that there was a slow leakage of aqueous humour after removal of the splinter. As a result the eye would have became flattened and iris tissue, because it is soft and pliable, would have become trapped in the wound and plugged it, like a curtain billowing into an open window. The price of all this would be a dilated, fixed pupil which would inevitably be distorted where the iris stuck to the wound site; this fits reasonably well with the appearance of Nelson's sightless eye.

Splinters are not usually clean so they tend to introduce bugs into the eye and of course there were no antibiotics in those days. Since the splinter had cut a long groove in Nelson's forehead, gone through his brow and lid and then into the eye, it may have been cleaner than most. However, it is likely that there was some infection in the eye and inflammation would explain the long period of pain following the injury. Nelson was very dismissive of his eye injury, as he was of all his injuries. Back in London at a later date, by which time he had lost an arm as well as having a sightless eye, when he was requested to visit military surgeons for an eye examination prior to the award of a pension, he said, 'Oh! this is only for an eye: in a few days I shall come for an arm: and in a little time longer, God knows, most probably for a leg.'

It should be said that there is a view held by some historians and ophthalmologists that Nelson's eye injury was not quite what was reported. Certainly his vision was lost but the injury may not have been as severe as the military surgeons were led to believe. Ophthalmologists have been convinced, on the basis of a portrait painted well before his injury, that there was scarring to his right eye even then. The scarring was not from an injury but was likely to have been a *pterygium*. This is a growth of opaque scar tissue from the conjunctiva and episclera over the cornea causing clouding and loss of vision.

The development of a pterygium is associated with excessive sunlight. Northern Europeans exposed to the sun in deserts or tropical seas are particularly prone to this problem. Ever since he was a young boy, Nelson had spent most of his time at sea, particularly in tropical waters. The implication is that, as Nelson received a pension for the loss of sight in his right eye, it was in his interests to play down the pterygium and play up the eye wound with the military board. To be fair to Nelson, he did receive the severe eye wound at the siege of Calvi as described above, but some question must remain about whether he would have had much sight in the right eye regardless of the injury.

The eye injury, as was the case with his other injuries, had little effect on his career and in one notable battle, it might be considered as being to his advantage. At the Battle of Copenhagen, Nelson's ships were to attack a line of enemy ships protected by their own shore batteries. The battle was fierce and it was difficult for Nelson's commander-in-chief to see who was getting the best of it. The commander-in-chief had had enough and signalled retreat, but when the signal was reported to Nelson, he said, 'I have only one eye – I have a right to be blind sometimes.' Then he put his telescope up to the blind right eye and said, 'I really do not see the signal!' Nelson's ships pressed on and, by means of his blind eye, a major victory was won.

PAINTERS

Going blind is a handicap to musicians, a crisis for writers and poets, but the end of the road for most artists. However, there have been many artists whose defective sight, in one form or another, has influenced their life and their painting. I will mention a few of these painters.

El Greco

Domenico Theotocopuli (1541–1614), better known as El Greco, was the product of an interesting mix of styles and cultures. Born in Crete, he trained in Italy (probably as a student of Titian) and worked for the bulk of his life in Spain. At first he painted entirely in the Venetian style, which is hardly surprising given his background, but with maturity Spanish influences crept into his work and thus evolved a style that is unique.

His Spanish home city was Toledo where he obtained many of the commissions that contributed to the impressive amount of work he completed during his lifetime. Sixteenth-century Spain was powerful, rich and committed to the Counter-Reformation, which revitalized the Catholic Church but also brought misery in the form of the notorious Inquisition. The Church, however, brought a great deal of work to El Greco in the form of paintings and altarpieces. Characteristics of El Greco's paintings are that his figures often have elongated heads, they seem to lean a little to the right, their fingers can be excessively long if pointing in a certain direction and, for want of better words, they have a wispy unreal quality about them.

These characteristics of El Greco's figures became more distinctive as he grew older until you could almost call the figures El Greco people. It is said that his characteristic style is an exaggeration of a technique adopted from Tintoreto and other Italian masters with the intention of creating in his figures a sense of unreality next to godliness. There are others who have argued that the El Greco style may be due less to a deliberately adopted technique than to an uncorrected astigmatism which became worse as he grew older. Astigmatism is, as has been noted in chapter 2, due to the cornea (and sometimes the lens) having optical irregularities and not being optically perfect for bending light, with the result that images are focused more strongly in one direction than another. Too many irregularities and there will be distortions sufficient to have visual consequences.

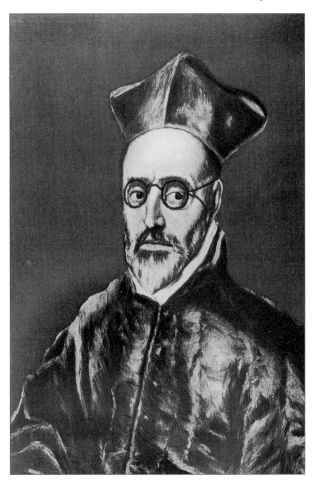

Figure 5.2 Detail of a painting by El Greco of Cardinal Guevara,
the Spanish Inquisitor General. He wears glasses.
(*With permission from the Metropolitan Museum of Art, New York*)

Whether or not El Greco had progressive astigmatism is open to debate and was a matter of considerable argument throughout the twentieth century among ophthalmologists as well as art critics. Whatever the facts of the matter, they do not detract from the fact that he was an original artist of the highest calibre. One device that El Greco used frequently was to give his religious figures and saints divergent squints (see chapter 4), these were meant to portray a sense of heavenly euphoria.

My own favourite El Greco painting is of Cardinal Guevara. The cardinal was Inquisitor General, and El Greco painted him sitting in his magnificent robes. The face is long and lengthened further by a pointed beard; his nose is also long (Figure 5.2). These are not the features of a kindly man; he is a man of power and it is difficult to imagine many sinners escaping from his courts with just a caution! Adding to the overall effect are the glasses he wears tied by string round his ears in a style of the time. The glasses don't look odd but enhance the cardinal's stern appearance. Was it the painter or the cardinal who insisted on the glasses being worn for the portrait? El Greco influenced many other painters, including Velázquez and Paul Cézanne, whom we consider next.

Paul Cézanne

Paul Cézanne (1839–1906) was one of the best of the Impressionist artists and can be considered as the first of the Post-Impressionists. His work is highly individual and I have chosen him because he is my favourite Impressionist artist. I could, however, equally have focused here on any of several Impressionist painters since, like Cézanne, Monet, the 'father' of Impressionism, Pissarro, Braque, Matisse and Degas all shared the same impediment: they were all short-sighted, or myopic (see chapter 2). So many of the Impressionist painters were short-sighted that Impressionism has been called by some the style of the poor-sighted painter.

That is very dismissive of a movement in art which broke down old barriers and conventions and led the way towards modern art. The criticism does contain some grain of truth, however, without diminishing in any way the contributions made by these great artists. Short-sighted people, as has been noted before, have larger than normal eyes and without glasses can see close to, but distance is a blur. Uncorrected, the disability has an influence on personality and preference (for information on this, see *The World through Blunted Sight* by Patrick Trevor-Roper). Myopes tend to have difficulties with sports, and outdoor activities such as hill-walking to see a view are a waste of time. Their preference is more likely to be for activities such as reading, writing and the like. In times gone by, when glasses were considered to be unmanly or unladylike, short-sighted people were to a great extent isolated in their infirmity and tended to become 'loners'.

Paul Cézanne had some of these characteristics, being, among other things, a great writer of letters. He was a loner and often lonely in the physical sense; he did not make friends easily but those he did make were extremely important to him. He was thought by many, rather unkindly, to be an ill-tempered recluse. Cézanne put up with his short-sightedness and would not put on glasses, which he thought were very 'vulgar things'. As a result his paintings have characteristics of the myope's world, the world he saw. The detail in his paintings is all in the foreground and his backgrounds are often non-existent or a blur. He loved to paint faces, bodies (particularly bathers) and still life. He did paint landscapes, but they tend to lack detail, unless there are prominent objects in the foreground.

Cézanne suffered from diabetes and the visual deterioration he experienced in later life may well have been due to the onset of diabetic eye disease (see chapter 4). However, his painting did not deteriorate with his failing vision, and the last part of his life might be called his most influential. It was during this period that some of his most distinguished works were produced. Paul Cézanne said of himself at that time, 'I am becoming more clear-sighted before nature, but with me the realization of my senses is always painful.' (Richard Kendall, *Cezanne by himself*. See Further Reading.) Undoubtedly he was referring in part to his weakening eyesight.

I love Cézanne's colours, which bear little relationship to true colour balance – it is all his own. Myopes have a preference towards browns and reds at the expense of blues. Blue hues are short wavelength and are bent more by the optics of the eye than reds, so they will not be favoured by the bigger myopic eye. Blue is a prominent colour in very few of Cézanne's pictures, most being dominated by browns, reds, bold greens and some yellow. The yellow chair in *Mrs Cézanne in a Yellow Armchair* is orange-brown to me and his skies, as in *Near the Pool at the Jas de Bouffan* and *The Great Pine* are all violets and purples. Would his *Boy in a Red Waistcoat* have been such an attractive subject to Cézanne if he was wearing blue?

Sir Joshua Reynolds

Joshua Reynolds (1723–92) was the greatest and most acclaimed portrait painter of his day. His paintings of the well-to-do, nobility and royalty hang in the best galleries and stately homes in the country. Although he does not give us a true picture of eighteenth-century life in Britain (that is more Holbein's province), he does give us an insight into the gentry of that time.

Both Reynolds' eyes began to fail in around 1789, probably because of internal leakage of blood into his eyes which obscured the retina and also caused internal retinal damage. His doctors did not know, until after his death, what was wrong with his eyes, other than thinking he didn't have cataracts. Reynolds feared the worst and thought he might have some kind of cancer. He was subjected to all sorts of horrible treatments, including leeches, blistering and vast amounts of mercury. To cap it all, he was advised to stop painting to save what vision he had left. Not surprisingly he did not survive more than a year.

POETS AND WRITERS

Writing this book I try to imagine how difficult it would be to be visually impaired and do the same – there are so many visual tasks to perform. I also remind myself that story making and telling are far older than the written word, being the device of minstrels and travellers.

Homer

Homer lived sometime around 700 to 1000 BC and is the earliest Greek poet whose work has survived. His two works, the *Iliad* and the *Odyssey*, are in the form of epic poems which tell the story of the war between the Greeks and Trojans and events thereafter, a war that took place several hundred years before Homer was born. Little is known about Homer except that he was blind, although we cannot even take that for granted. The evidence for his blindness is flimsy and based on one line about himself which says in effect, that he is a blind man.

Other evidence is extremely tenuous and stems largely from the absence from his verse of very many visual images and colour words. The experts may say that there are few of these images when compared with work by a sighted poet, but an example is 'rosy-fingered dawn', which is pretty good for a presumed blind man!

John Milton

John Milton (1608–74) was a poet from the time of the English Civil War who was a strong supporter of Oliver Cromwell and the Parliamentarian side against King Charles I. When he wasn't embroiled in the dangerous politics of the time, he composed poems and sonnets that place him among England's greats.

Milton had poor eyesight and eventually went blind when only 44 years old – 'Vaunting aloud, but racked with deep despair.' It is not known exactly what brought about his blindness but glaucoma, and alternatively retinal detachment, have been considered by the current-day experts. These conditions are as likely as anything else and their onset fits with Milton's descriptions of his failing eyesight. Another suggestion that has been put forward is that Milton had a slowly developing cancer of the brain (the pituitary gland to be exact), which, as it grew, encroached on his vision.

Many quotes in his subsequent works refer to blindness and its isolation – 'To sit in darkness here/Hatching vain empires' – but this was a period of some stability that he had not had in his younger years and was also the period when he created his very best work, *Paradise Lost.* He did not sleep very well and worked on the poem during the night. When the structure of a few lines was in a format with which he was satisfied he would get his daughter Anna to write them down for him. Slowly, ever so slowly, the blind man organized his thoughts and created his masterpiece.

William Wordsworth

> I wandered lonely as a cloud
> That floats on high o'er vales and hills,
> When all at once I saw a crowd,
> A host, of golden daffodils ...

The Lakeland poet William Wordsworth (1770–1850) wrote 'Daffodils' and so created some of the best-known lines in British poetry. He may have seen 'a host, of golden daffodils' and enjoyed the beauty of the Lake District, but his sight was not all it might have been and became much worse in later years. His eyes were itchy and troublesome because they were subject to inflammation and scarring – he had trachoma (see chapter 4).

Wordsworth spent his early years in Paris, travelled in Europe a little and spent a considerable time in London. Although trachoma is an eye disease we associate with poor hygiene and the dry conditions of the Middle Eastern countries, he never travelled that far. Wordsworth caught his trachoma in a European city, probably London, because this was the time at the end of the eighteenth century and the beginning of the nineteenth when European wars tended to spill out of Europe and take on a world-wide aspect. The medical significance was that European soldiers and sailors exported diseases like mumps and measles wherever they went and returned home with an abundance of exotic diseases, one of which was trachoma.

Many of the poor parts of European cities at that time were effectively cesspools, and London was top of the list for filth and squalor; many areas were hardly fit to live in and the perfect places for the transmission of the infective trachoma agent. During the Napoleonic wars, France invaded Egypt and where the French went, the English had to follow. Many of those troops who returned from this conflict had trachoma and once they were back in England, the eye disease reached epidemic proportions in the crowded, poorer parts of London. There was such alarm in the capital that funds were made available to set up a hospital that would specialize in eye diseases. This was the beginning of Moorfields Eye Hospital (see also chapter 3).

Trachoma is particularly unpleasant in the Middle East because the dry, dusty climate makes the eyes even more itchy and sore; it stands to reason therefore that the sooty, unpleasant air of nineteenth-century cities can't have been very kind to trachoma eyes either. The damp, clean air of the Lake District must have added to that region's attractions for Wordsworth. Here he settled with his wife and sister, supplementing his income by holding the post of 'distributor of stamps for Westmorland'. Life was not entirely idyllic: the infective organism was most severe in his eyelids and when it was particularly bad he could do little, certainly not write anything. This fuelled his growing frustrations and helped to dampen his creativity. Towards the end of his life he was made Poet Laureate, but would Wordsworth have been even more creative had he not had trachoma?

James Joyce

In the late 1960s some friends and I travelled, mostly on foot, across Scotland to a small town called Alloa in Clackmannanshire to see a film version of James Joyce's *Ulysses* which had been banned from the cinema screens elsewhere in that country (so much for the Swinging Sixties). You might think that we were high-brow intellectuals or, at the very least, film buffs. In fact we were just a motley crew of teenagers who knew nothing of Joyce or his major work, and we definitely would not have made the trip if we had known the least thing about Joyce's writing. We were driven on by faulty logic and teenage hormones: if it was banned from so many cinemas, it must be really dirty!

As it was, most of us slept through the long film and those who had the stamina to stay awake after such a long journey felt thoroughly cheated. 'Far too much acting and little in the way of stripping' and 'No action, just talking' were examples of the range of critical evaluations expressed later in the pub where we spent the last of our money that should have given us a roof over our heads for the night to come. Joyce (1882–1941) was used to his work being vilified in his lifetime, but now *Ulysses* can be read by all and appreciated along with his other novels such as *Dubliners* and *Finnegans Wake* as major contributions to western literature (Figure 5.3).

I must admit I still find *Ulysses* very hard going and *Finnegans Wake* almost impossible to read. Joyce was a perfectionist and struggled with every phrase and sentence in his major works. Uncorrected, short-sighted people make interesting painters as, for example, with the Impressionists (see Cézanne, already discussed), but uncorrected or otherwise they are in their element as writers. James Joyce was short-sighted and had all the schoolboy problems of having to wear what in his case were rather thick and unsightly glasses. He was very introspective. How much was that introspection aggravated by his weak sight and the isolation that can bring to some children?

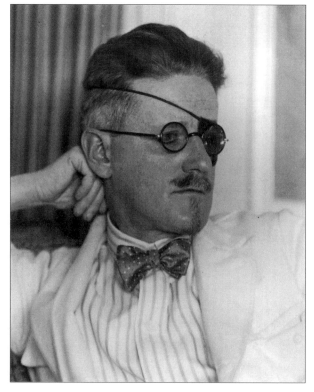

Figure 5.3   Photograph of James Joyce taken in 1926.
(*Commerce Graphics Inc., USA*)

As a young man, Joyce developed a condition called iritis (an inflammation of the iris and surrounding tissues) in both his eyes. The bouts of
inflammation were recurrent and severe, and consequently they triggered
glaucoma (see secondary glaucoma in chapter 4) which required surgery to
lower the increased pressure and relieve some of the symptoms. His eyesight,
poor enough to begin with, gradually deteriorated (despite no less than ten
eye operations) so that, towards the end of his life, he could no longer read
normal print.

I find Joyce hard going because he was less interested in the plot of a
novel than in words themselves. His work became progressively more
obscure as his sight deteriorated; the two facts may not be entirely inter-
dependent but it does seem likely that this man, who seems not to have
liked himself very much, became even less happy with passing time and
failing vision. His escape in his later works, such as *Finnegans Wake*, was
in complex word play and images far from the real world. The opening
lines of a book are often said to capture its essence. The opening of *Finnegans
Wake* is: 'riverrun, past Eve and Adam's, from swerve of shore to bend of

bay, brings us by a commodius vicus of recirculation back to Howth Castle and Environs' – and, for me, it doesn't get any easier.

James Thurber

James Thurber (1894–1961) was an entirely different type of person from Joyce, being a humorous man who wrote humorous books. Perhaps he is not as well known as once he was, but his books are still gems. He drew excellent cartoons and was quick-witted; once, after picking up the phone and dialling, he is quoted as saying, 'Well, if I called the wrong number, why did you answer the phone?'

Thurber wrote *The Secret Life of Walter Mitty* about a man who is harried and henpecked by his wife, and whose only means of escape is to enter into fantasy daydreams in which he is the brave hero. The comedian Danny Kaye played Walter Mitty in the screen version of the book, a classic film which has led to the expression 'Walter Mitty character' finding a place in common English usage.

James Thurber is mentioned in this book because he had poor vision for most of his life as a result of a terrible accident when he was a child. During a game of cowboys and Indians, his brother fired an arrow from his bow and hit him in the eye. Thurber was doubly unlucky because he not only lost the injured eye, he also developed a sympathetic inflammation in the good eye. This is a rare but devastating condition that can occur after a severe injury to one eye when an inflammation develops not only in the injured eye but also in the good eye. The inflammation occurs because the immune system can be stimulated after major eye damage to produce antibodies against all eye tissue, damaged or otherwise.

Fear of this sympathetic inflammation in the good eye leads eye surgeons to remove a badly damaged eye if all chance of retaining some sight in it has been lost. Thurber had to spend the rest of his life with his body trying to reject his good eye. The result was repeated bouts of inflammation and deteriorating sight by the time he was in his forties. He continued to work on his stories and his comic pictures under the most difficult circumstances, drawing larger and larger cartoons to compensate for his failing vision. When he descended into blindness he continued to work by means of dictation. 'A blind man benefits by lack of distractions' was a typical Thurber statement.

CLASSICAL COMPOSERS AND MUSICIANS

Of the composers with eye problems selected here, two had cataract problems and one was treated for cataract (which he may not have had), and they serve to illustrate what a major problem this was for the elderly in days gone by. Each of these three went blind late in life, whereas the fourth composer discussed had to live with blindness for much of his life.

Johann Sebastian Bach

J. S. Bach (1685–1750) came from a family of very skilled musicians living in northern Germany. He himself had a massive family of twenty children, of whom several were talented musicians in their own right. Bach was a good singer, an excellent organist and a composer of true genius, creating concertos (of which the Brandenberg series is perhaps the best known), copious numbers of cantatas, masses of organ works and hundreds of shorter works. He had a particular skill in writing for organ, piano and choirs.

Bach had only modest eyesight but went completely blind a year or so before his death when he had a sudden loss of vision and complained bitterly of pain behind the eyes. It is hard to say what the problem was, but he may have had a complaint that restricted the arterial supply of blood to the eyes. An oculist by the name of 'Chevalier' Taylor was recommended to him (see the history of ophthalmology in chapter 3). Dr Samuel Johnson, the dictionary writer, who had eye problems of his own, said of Taylor that he was 'an incidence of how far impudence will carry ignorance'.

Taylor was a charlatan who had built up a considerable reputation in Europe as an eye doctor but, even for those days, most of his remedies were pretty grim. The majority did no good at all but others were actually dangerous, and true to form he subjected Bach to cuts in the eyes, mercury treatment and bleeding. Taylor treated the composer for cataracts, which he may have had, but these would not have led to his sudden blindness and are not associated with pain. The quack oculist not only diagnosed the cause of the blindness incorrectly but also subjected Bach to extra pain and infection. Bach had a truly miserable time in his last year, due, in great part, to his eye problems. The cuts and mercury treatment produced a chronic inflammation within and around the eyes which brought him considerable discomfort.

George Frideric Handel

George Frideric Handel (1685–1759) was born in Halle, Germany but most of his working life was spent in London and he had British citizenship. He was a proficient player of many instruments, but was particularly talented on the harpsichord and a most gifted organ player. He set up a Royal Academy of Music in London which was an opera company specializing in Italian-style opera. However, Gay's *Beggar's Opera* fired the public's enthusiasm for works in English and George Handel's response to this trend led to one of his greatest works, the *Messiah* oratorio, which contains the well-known 'Hallelujah Chorus'. He is also known for his superbly melodious music including the *Water Music* and the anthems written for the coronation of George II, which have been a major part of coronations ever since.

By all accounts Handel was a big, hearty man who had a huge appetite for both food and alcohol. After extraordinary financial ups and downs in his life, Handel spent his last years as a wealthy man. It is ironic, therefore, that this period was associated with failing sight leading to blindness. Handel and Bach were born in the same year (1685), they both had eye problems and unfortunately they both had the same oculist, the notorious Chevalier Taylor. Handel went completely blind from his fully developed cataracts in 1743 and the oculist performed a needling operation on him, attempting to push the opaque lens out of the pathway of vision. At least this time, unlike with Bach, Taylor was treating the correct condition, but his procedure was to no avail because Handel remained completely blind. As has been mentioned in chapter 3, it was at about this time that Jacques Daviel developed a cataract operation that involved the complete removal of the lens. It would prove to be far more successful, but only if performed by skilled hands, hands that Chevalier Taylor certainly did not seem to have.

Franz Liszt

The composer Franz Liszt (1811–1886) was a sickly child who nearly died following a smallpox vaccination at six years of age. Edward Jenner had recently introduced the technique of injecting the less virulent cowpox virus to prevent smallpox, but, probably because the doses were neither standardized nor sterilized, the procedure was nearly the death of young Liszt. Despite his sickly youth, Liszt grew up to be a fine young man and his considerable talent on the piano elevated him to international fame. He produced copious numbers of musical compositions and it is chiefly as a composer that we know of him today, but in his own time this achievement was less important: his reputation was based on being the most outstanding pianist in the world.

Liszt was in constant demand and spent most of his life travelling around Europe from one concert venue to another, remaining active right up to his death. He had adoring fans who would mob his concerts in much the same way as happens with pop stars today. He also exhibited what can be see as pop star characteristics in that he was reputed to drink far more than was good for him and he was very much a ladies' man. In his later years, unfortunately, he had numerous chronic ailments, one of the most devastating for him being the relentless development of cataracts, first in his left eye and then in the right. In his final year his vision was so poor that he sometimes needed help eating. Additionally Liszt developed a severe swelling of his eyelids (blepharitis) which resulted in his eyes watering continuously.

You might expect that, with the eye problems and the host of other illnesses, Liszt would take things easy. In fact, the opposite was the case and his last year was one of his busiest. He had to be led to his piano for concerts and he adjusted his playing style to compensate for his poor vision. The visual decline did not take the edge off his playing; it is recorded that in his last years Liszt played the piano extremely well and still captivated his audiences. As might be expected, only in composition and music reading did he struggle.

The story of the later years of Franz Liszt moves me in two ways. The first is through my admiration for his tenacity to be the best and remain the best despite the problems and handicaps that were placed in his way. The second is through the realization of how devastating cataracts were in those days. Now a cataract operation can be done in a day ward and is considered a relatively simple procedure. Liszt, with all his fame and fortune, had the pick of eye surgeons in Europe and went to the best. However, despite having the pick of the crop, he still chose visual handicap rather than endure the hazards and pain of the nineteenth-century operating table. The loss of vision became so extreme that Liszt finally agreed to have his cataracts removed, but sadly he died a few weeks before the scheduled operation.

Frederick Delius

Frederick Delius (1862–1934) as a young man was wild and bohemian. It was during his early adult life that he contracted syphilis, which at that time, before the advent of antibiotics, could have very serious consequences indeed. Conventional medical treatment in the nineteenth and early twentieth century traditionally consisted of mercury-based concoctions which had many awful side-effects and there was little clear evidence that they had any real action on the disease itself. Later bismuth treatments and then arsenic compounds were introduced, which were far more useful and had fewer side-effects. Unfortunately Delius didn't use any of the better conventional treatments but relied on homeopathy, which did nothing to counteract the full ravages of this terrible disease.

Complications in the later stages of syphilis include neurological disturbances and blindness. Delius had considerable pain in his eyes, his vision deteriorated and, although he only went completely blind in 1922, he was severely visually handicapped for much of his life. Of course, blindness was not his only disability: he also had frequent bouts of stomach cramp, his joints grew progressively more painful so that he had difficulty walking and, in the later years, his body wasted to almost nothing.

Delius had a quick, active and creative mind trapped in an ever-deteriorating body. He bore his afflictions well on the whole, although in his last few years he did became more frustrated and demanding. Delius was aided greatly by Eric Fenby who wrote for him and no doubt took the brunt of some of his outbursts. It must be very hard to be gifted and not able to give full rein to those gifts. Delius's music is well known for its atmospheric and dream-like qualities. Perhaps, in his music, there was an escape from the shackles of his failing health and deteriorating eyesight.

POPULAR SINGERS AND MUSICIANS

There is a large gap in this section because I have not included jazz musicians. This is due to my own ignorance and personal taste, and also the sheer abundance of blind and partially sighted jazz and blues players, including on a single page of a book I consulted on jazz performers, Blind Blake, Blind Willie McTell, Blind Garry Davies, Blind Boy Fuller and Blind Sonny Terry! I take comfort in the fact that two of my four chosen singers and musicians are honoured in this and many other jazz books, although they seem to fit more readily into the popular music scene.

When I asked my jazz-enthusiast friends the question as to why so many jazz and blues musicians were blind or poorly sighted, of course the answer was obvious. If you were brought up in a poor African-American family in the early part of the twentieth century and on top of this handicap you also had poor vision or no vision at all, what else could you do to make a living?

Ray Charles

Most of us remember a song and an artist who really influenced the type of popular music we liked most of all. For me, as a teenager in the early 1960s, the artist was Ray Charles (born 1930) and the song was a blues/rock-and-roll number called 'What'd I Say!' It was my introduction to rhythm and blues, a type of music I still love, even though I never quite got to grips with ethnic blues music or jazz. My close schoolfriend Matt Carruthers lived in a railway cottage opposite our school and often we would sneak away and play this record, among others, on Matt's record player. The record had been a minor hit in 1959 in Britain, but a major top ten hit in America. Ray Charles was never as popular in Britain as in the USA, where he is high in their rock-and-roll hall of fame, a well-deserved position in my opinion because his music had a huge influence on many of the 1960s bands on both sides of the Atlantic.

Ray Charles had a number one hit in the USA and the UK with 'I Can't Stop Loving You' in 1962, which was around the time I first started to listen to him. I only knew his music from records up until this time, so I had quite a shock when I became aware that this vibrant rock-and-roll, blues and ballad singer/pianist was blind. He had not been blind all his life, having lost his vision more or less completely only when he was six. It seems likely that Ray Charles (originally Ray Charles Robinson) had childhood glaucoma (congenital glaucoma, see chapter 4), a fortunately rare condition which is difficult to treat nowadays, but was visually fatal for a child born in the 1930s.

Ray Charles never really had a chance to have his vision saved. His mother was too poor to have him seen by a specialist, although she did later have the courage to send him to a special school for the blind. In his book *Brother Ray*, which includes his extremely frank memories of going blind, he said:

> Images began to blur, and I saw less and less. When I woke up, my little eyes were tight shut as a door, crusted over and so sticky that my eye lids were matted together. Sometimes Mama took a damp cloth and gently mopped around my eyes. After five or ten minutes, I'd slowly start blinking and adjusting to the morning light. But soon my horizons grew shorter and shorter. Faraway distances were fading. I was like a guy who stands on top of a mountain and one week sees fifteen miles off, the next week only ten miles, the third week only five. At first I could still make out large forms, then only colours, then only night from day.

At blind school, Ray received the education he otherwise might not have had, but also he was taught how to play the piano. His piano playing was great but his voice was superb. In a rock-and-roll song, a blues number or a ballad, his skill was to fill the number with passion, pain and sentiment. He has been called the father of soul music and that is a title that has been well earned. However, he also had a dark side and that was heroin; all his life he seems to have had a fight with drugs, which has brought major lows into his life. 'Take These Chains from My Heart and Set Me Free' was one of his hit records which has more meaning if placed in the context of his lifestyle.

Stevie Wonder

Stevie Wonder is one of the glittering stars of Tamla Motown and was born completely blind in 1950. He had his first US number one single, 'Fingertips', when he was only 13 years old, by which time he was able to sing like an angel, and play harmonica, piano and drums. A child genius of the pop world who managed to become a great performer and was also an innovator, Stevie Wonder was fascinated by electronic music and helped to set popular musical trends. However, he also managed by pure talent to be at a level above any passing fashion.

Towards the end of the 1970s, Stevie Wonder became a spokesman and activist for numerous good causes and political pressure groups for change. He was a particularly prominent voice in the campaign to have a day dedicated to the murdered civil rights leader Martin Luther King. In fact one of his best-known songs, 'Happy Birthday', released in the UK in 1981, was part of this campaign to commemorate King's birthday.

Recently Stevie Wonder has become associated with research work where the intention is to develop a microchip or diode to be inserted into the retina to provide artificial vision. I believe he has put himself forward as a candidate for at least one such research programme. Artificial vision has considerable potential for the future, but as yet the visual results are feeble (for more, see chapter 7).

David Bowie

David Jones was born in south London in 1947 and when he became set on a singing career, he changed his name to David Bowie to avoid confusion with Davy Jones of the Monkees. Bowie is one of the big international stars of popular music that Britain is fortunate to produce every now and again, whose fame is measured in decades, not months. He performed in groups in the 1960s, came to fame in the 1970s, became a major international superstar in the 1980s and remained at the pinnacle of pop success in the 1990s.

Bowie initiated many new trends and his over-the-top character Ziggy Stardust was the forerunner of the glam-rock fashion that so dominated British popular music in the 1970s. Bowie is not just a singer and writer of interesting songs; he is also a performer. His performances involved incredible costumes and fantastic make-up, particularly around his eyes, and he created a series of *alter egos* of which Ziggy Stardust is but one, although undoubtedly the most famous. As might be expected he has an enthusiasm for acting and has starred in a number of films, some splendid, others less so. David Bowie was and is a controversial figure who, for example, announced publicly his bisexuality at a time when such things were not done even by pop stars.

In recent years Bowie has become a more conservative dresser, but he could not be considered in any way to have a conservative appearance. Everything about him is striking. He has an angular face with boyish good looks which survive even now he is in his fifties. But why have I included David Bowie in this section of the book? If he has any visual problems, I must confess that I know nothing about them. My reason for including him is because, of all his striking features, the most striking are his eyes.

When I look at pictures of David Bowie I am drawn to his eyes; one is piercingly blue while the other is a greenish-brown. The difference between the two eyes is even more prominent because the pupil of the greenish-brown eye usually seems, in most of the pictures I have seen, to be larger than that of the blue eye. Technically the term for this condition is *iris hetero-chromia*. As mentioned in chapter 1, the basis of eye colour is still poorly understood, but it seems to be determined by the presence of the pigment melanin in cells called melanocytes which are present in the stroma of the iris. Melanin is responsible for hair and skin colour as well as eye colour. The melanocytes of a blue iris have less melanin in them than those of a green iris, whereas the melanocytes of a brown iris have even more melanin than the green.

There are minute differences in eye colour in many people but few have as marked a difference between the two eyes as David Bowie. Eye colour becomes established after we are born, through melanin formation, and in people with heterochromia the melanin production continues for a longer period in one eye than the other, whereas for the rest of us it stops more or less at the same time in both eyes. David Bowie seems to have a fascination with 'out of this world' events, space travel and aliens, and many of his record titles, lyrics and film roles reflect this: 'Space Oddity', 'Life on Mars', 'The Rise and Fall of Ziggy Stardust and the Spiders from Mars', 'Scary Monsters', 'Starman', 'Loving the Alien' and 'Earthling' are just a few of his titles. One of his best-known film roles was as a stranded alien in *The Man who Fell to Earth* (1976). I wonder if Bowie's preoccupation with difference and other-worldliness has anything to do with his having the rare condition of iris heterochromia?

STATESMEN AND POLITICIANS

Is a statesman someone in politics you admire and a politician someone you don't? Or is it that a statesman is a politician who has been dead for more than 10 years? There were many for me to choose from, as, perhaps surprisingly, eye problems have been rife in the past and present worlds of politics, but with scant regard for balance I mention two past presidents of the USA and two current Labour cabinet ministers.

Abraham Lincoln

By all accounts US president Abraham Lincoln (1809–65) was a startling looking fellow for a statesman and politician: long and skinny with huge hands and feet, and sporting a mop of uncontrolled hair which was stuffed into a preposterously tall hat. Some doctors have suggested that Lincoln had a condition called *Marfan's syndrome*; certainly he had the physical features that are associated with the disease and Marfan patients often have weak eyesight.

Abraham Lincoln was long-sighted and had very poor vision in one eye due to what has been described as a 'lazy eye' (see chapter 4). He may have had an untreated squint and, as we know, the brain suppresses vision in the squinting eye, making it lazy and the vision poor or absent. If he did have Marfan's syndrome, the explanation for the poor vision might be quite different. Marfan patients have problems with the elastic tissue that is found in the skin and all over the body. In the eye, elastic tissue is the main component of the threads called zonules which hold the lens in place (see chapter 1) and in a complication of Marfan's syndrome the threads can break and the lens become dislocated. If Lincoln had a dislocated lens in one eye, his vision would be very poor, but this is mere speculation. It is part of American folklore that his first and favourite spectacles cost him the princely sum of 38 cents.

Harry Truman

Harry S. Truman (1884–1972), president of the USA from 1945 to 1953, always had very poor eyesight which was a handicap to him all his life. He was a small man, distinguished by his thick 'bottle end' glasses, who steered the USA through the last few months of the Second World War and through the troubled peace. The Korean War was also during his period in office. I think he was one among several great statesmen of the time, the others including Winston Churchill and Charles De Gaulle. Truman had determination, lots of drive and a way of getting what he wanted even when the odds were stacked against him; in the USA, someone they call 'a winner'.

I like the story of Truman's medical for the army, which underlines his determination to succeed where others might give up. In his youth he wanted to join the services, but, of course, when he applied for officer's training at West Point, he failed the eye test. It was a bitter disappointment, but it did not put him off. He became involved in the local territorial army and, when he enlisted for active service during the First World War, he was better prepared. He managed to sneak through the eye test by previously doing his homework and memorizing the Snellen Eye Chart (see chapters 2 and 3). He obtained a commission and reached the rank of captain, spending the war on the battlefields of France.

Gordon Brown

The cofounder of 'New Labour', Gordon Brown is a powerful figure in current UK politics. He was born in 1951, the son of a Scottish minister, and went to university at the tender age of 16. I first heard of him when he became Student Rector of Edinburgh University, at a time when a captain of industry or a popular personality held the post, usually as a figurehead. Gordon Brown was a very controversial figure and a thorn in the side of what was then a very stuffy university establishment. I was studying at Glasgow University at this time and what Gordon Brown might try next was a matter of considerable student interest.

What I didn't know then was that Gordon Brown had lost the sight of one eye and was only partially sighted in the other. He suffered a total retinal detachment in his left eye and a partial detachment in his right as a result of an injury sustained while playing rugby for his school. He underwent a series of operations which succeeded only in giving him some vision in the eye with the partial detachment; the other was visually useless. It must be said that his detachments had probably been there for some months before treatment, and also that the treatment available in the 1960s was not nearly as advanced as it is now; these factors made his chances of good vision being restored fairly remote.

Brown had to spend time with his eyes covered and he was told not to study, and as a result he fell behind in his university work. What might have been a handicap to others was only a nuisance to him, and not only did he ultimately romp through his studies, he also became a leading figure in university politics. Gordon Brown ended up with a first-class honours in history and a research doctorate, and was a very active Rector of the University to boot. Following a stint in Scottish television, he became MP for a Scottish constituency. He has had two opportunities to stand for the leadership of the Labour Party and both times has spurned the chance. Along with Tony Blair, Brown had a great deal to do with shaping New Labour and he can take considerable credit for Labour's massive electoral victory in 1997, after which he became Chancellor of the Exchequer.

Being such a powerful figure, it is not surprising that Brown has his critics, who unfortunately are not just restricted to the opposition benches and the press. He is considered by some to be unsmiling, perhaps a little too intellectual, too intense and rather gloomy. I understand from what has been written about him that he likes to keep his private life very private. It may be that his natural reticence works against him in these circumstances, allowing his shyness to be misinterpreted as aloofness. How much his damaged eyesight has moulded his character over the years can only be guessed at but, even for someone as clever as Gordon Brown, life for a politician with dim vision must be tough at times. Kenneth Clarke, the previous Conservative Chancellor, said when attacking Brown in the Commons that he had a 'most impressive pile of books'. Gordon Brown is well known for rattling off all sorts of statistics to make his political points, but the books were not there for that reason. The vision in his good eye is so limited that he puts his notes on top of the books so that he can read them clearly.

David Blunkett

It must be difficult at times for Gordon Brown in the rough house that is politics, but it must be even worse for David Blunkett. Following Labour's victory in 1997, Blunkett was given the extremely difficult post of Secretary of State for Education and Employment – not a job for someone faint of heart and David Blunkett is anything but that. Blind from birth, Blunkett has shown the country that a blind man can take on the rough and tumble of modern-day politics and do far more than hold his own.

The optic nerves (see chapter 1) of David Blunkett's eyes did not form properly, so when he was born he had no vision at all. When he was very young, his parents, particularly his father, disregarded his blindness and treated him as if he were sighted. The young David Blunkett as a result knew no preconceived limits and felt no handicap: an invaluable start to life. At the age of four he went to a school for the blind as a boarder, which, for him, was not a happy experience. The loneliness he felt at the boarding school helped him develop a protective shell which at some times is a comfort and at other times a curse.

Blunkett was involved in politics initially in his native Sheffield and then became an MP. During his first few years as an MP, he used to make his way to the House of Commons from his flat in south London via the Underground, aided on this perilous route by his guide dog. One thing he didn't pick up during these early years, unlike most politicians, is the politician's smile – the smile they don't really mean. As a result of his blindness, David Blunkett has never learned to smile on cue, which, in many eyes no doubt, is to his credit.

I like the story of Blunkett's first full ministry meeting with the Prime Minister, Tony Blair. He got out his *Braille* papers, which had just been typed up on the brand new Braille machine bought specially from Sweden for his department, and ran his fingers over the indentations, only to find that they were gibberish. He managed to carry on and bluff it out, relying entirely on memory. When he got back to his department, he found that the new machine bought from Sweden only spoke Swedish! This is the kind of problem a sighted cabinet minister fortunately does not have to come up against. But David Blunkett has shown the world that blindness does not in any way debar you from a full and active life in politics.

SPORTS PERSONALITIES

Gordon Banks

One of soccer's legends and the outstanding English goalkeeper of the

1960s, Gordon Banks played in the England team that won the 1966 World Cup. He also played in the following World Cup of 1970 where, against Brazil, he made a save which ranks among the greatest of all time. Even Pelé, the Brazilian star whose perfect header Banks miraculously saved, said that it was the greatest save he had ever seen. Banks played most of his career with Leicester City and then later moved to Stoke, meanwhile winning 73 caps for England.

In 1972, Banks was driving home for Sunday lunch when he crashed head-on into an on-coming van. He was not wearing a seat belt and suffered injuries which included windscreen glass in his right eye. An ophthalmic surgeon operated on his eye, but although he was able to remove all the debris and repair the eye physically, the eye was functionally useless. At this point in his life Gordon Banks was probably one of the best-known people in Britain: Stoke had won the League Cup that year, a couple of years earlier Banks had been awarded an OBE and he was the current 'Footballer of the Year' and 'Sportsman of the Year'. After the car crash Banks felt that his life was in ruins.

In one way it was indeed in ruins: with only one eye, it was always going to be difficult to return to being a goalkeeper again, never mind one of the very best. No doubt going from being the number one at a sport to something not quite as good is the nightmare all sportsmen dread, but one of course that happens to them all in the end. Banks, however, was playing against Liverpool on Saturday, had his car crash on Sunday and that was it. From that position, it might be expected that he would give up entirely and just think that life was against him. He did have his black times, but he fought his way out of them and tried to get back to first-class goalkeeping.

The first problem for a one-eyed goalkeeper is the loss of binocular vision (see chapter 2) and the second is the loss of field of vision. Put simply he would not be as clearly aware of what was going on around him, particularly to the right. Not knowing exactly where he should stand in any situation and where exactly the ball was in flight would be considerable problems that needed to be solved. Banks worked hard at getting fit again and then worked even harder on his goalkeeping, but this was a slow process and neither Stoke nor he at that time was convinced he could return to anything like club class.

Banks had to get to grips with his more restricted monocular view of the football pitch, but his timing was off and he was missing shots he would have saved before his accident. This was not helped by the fact that he found it far more difficult to judge the speed of the ball when it was coming towards the goal. Banks played in friendly matches but didn't enjoy his football because he had the underlying fear that he would make a fool of himself. Confidence is very important to a goalkeeper. Stoke dropped him as a goalie and he took a job as coach to the youth players.

As time went by, Banks adjusted and began to improve in goal; by his standards he felt he was less than perfect, but now he could keep goal at a useful level. He was asked to join the Fort Lauderdale Strikers in the US league and took the job. He was a great success and was voted 'Goalkeeper of the Year'. After a two-year stint in the USA, he returned to England to become goalkeeper for Port Vale. He may not have recaptured the form of his World Cup days, but he had made it back to league standard. Not bad for a man who had only the sight of one eye and had thought his playing days were over.

Frank Bruno

Heavyweight boxer and one-time WBC world champion Frank Bruno's longest fight has been against eye problems. He is probably one of the best-known British boxers of current times and ranks alongside the likes of Henry Cooper in public affection. His professional boxing career very nearly never got off the ground because at the medical, required for his boxing licence, it was found that he was short-sighted in his right eye to the extent that the licence application was refused. Bruno was devastated, but then he heard of a pioneering operation called radial keratotomy (RK) that was being carried out only in Russia and South America. It is an operation where the surgeon makes cuts in the cornea to change its shape and thus counteract the short sight (see chapter 3). Bruno went to Bogotá for the treatment and a year or so later he was in the ring in his first professional fight.

Eye problems were to dog Frank's career and a second scare came not long after he fought Mike Tyson, unsuccessfully, for the world championship. During the course of a routine eye check-up, he was found to have developed a tear in the retina of his already problematical right eye. Again he thought his career might be at an end and there was an outcry in the press for him to retire. The furore was fuelled not only by a growing alarm about the dangers associated with the sport but also by a genuine affection for Bruno as a person. It was inaccurately reported that he had a retinal detachment and not a retinal tear; of the two, a tear is less serious. Both can be treated and will generally have a very satisfactory outcome. However, a retinal detachment would leave the tissue too weak to continue boxing, whereas a retinal tear, once repaired, does not leave the retina any weaker than it was before the damage. Bruno was able to have his retinal tear repaired by an operation that involves freezing the tear into place and he then regained his boxing licence.

Frank Bruno went on to gain the highest honours in his sport by becoming WBC heavyweight champion of the world in 1995 when he beat

Oliver McCall, but this was to be his high point. Unfortunately for the British boxer, Mike Tyson seemed to save his best fights for him and again he defeated Bruno. About a year later it turned out to be an eye specialist and not a boxer who gave him the final knock-out. It seems that the right eye had deteriorated to the extent that his specialist was quoted as saying, 'There is a risk he could be blinded in the eye if he steps into the ring again. He is in danger of getting a retinal detachment and there is no point exposing himself to that.'

I don't think anyone in medicine would recommend boxing as a sport that is good for either the eyes or the brain. Blows to the upper part of the head can overcome the defences that protect the eye (see chapter 1) and the eye physically distorts with the impact of the blow. The distortion brings stresses to the coats of the eye, particularly the most delicate inner coat, the retina. This can become detached over a period of time dependent on the number and severity of the blows. Some people's retinas are naturally poorly attached compared with those of the rest of the population, and it is these individuals who are vulnerable to retinal detachment as a result of boxing and other contact sports. Only a few boxers suffer retinal detachment, but that is a few too many.

Dennis Taylor

I used to play snooker with my Dad in our local social club. Snooker, for those who have never played it, is not the easy game it looks when you see the professionals on television. We were good enough to hit the right ball, but not good enough to pot it regularly. Our games would go on for ages: a red here and another one there, and on occasion a colour would go into the pocket after the potted red, or perhaps, once in a blue moon, another red and another colour would be sunk in sequence – that would be the talking point of the evening. Most of the people I know who play snooker enjoy the game at this level, and it is in stark contrast to the professionals who are so good.

The difficulty is that potting a ball depends on a myriad of different factors: the distance the cue ball is away from the one you want to pot (the object ball), the angle and distance between the ball and the pocket, how hard you strike the cue ball, the speed of the cushions, the smoothness of the cloth, what kind of spin you put on the cue ball, where the cue ball hits the object ball and a host of other variables all matter. In addition, you must be able to judge the 'weight' and 'direction' of the cue ball so that after the first pot is completed it is in an ideal position for the next pot. It is this latter part of the game that is beyond all but the very experienced and the very talented.

Among other things, good touch, good cueing and good vision (distance judgement and visual acuity) are vital for success in snooker. The very best players are instinctive but if their vision is off, this can make the difference between winning and losing in highly competitive games. The vision part of the game creates a problem for the short-sighted player. Wearing normal glasses means that, when the player looks down and along the cue, the shot is lined up looking not through the centre of the glasses where they are optically ideal, but way off centre where there is distortion. In addition, as was mentioned in chapter 3, glasses restrict your field of vision and some types of shot do require looking out of the 'corner' of the eye. Some players cope without using glasses, accepting that on long shots the pocket and the target ball will be a blur. Contact lenses can be the answer for short matches, but in the long professional tournaments, under the bright table lights and bright television lights, the lenses and eyes can dry out, causing irritation and oxygen starvation to the corneas.

Dennis Taylor is a snooker player of great skill who has been at the top of his profession for many years. He is short-sighted and in his time he has run into all the visual problems I have mentioned and a few more besides. He was born in Northern Ireland and became a professional snooker player in 1971. He played very well, but never quite managed to win the big tournaments. Things came to a head when, in 1979, he reached the final of the World Professional Championship at the Crucible in Sheffield. His opponent, Terry Griffiths, and he were neck and neck, reaching 15 frames all, but at this point it all went wrong for Taylor. His game collapsed completely, and Griffiths ended up the runaway victor by 24 frames to 16. Taylor was generous in defeat, rightly praising the skill of the winner, but he did not mention that his eyes were red raw. The intense light over the period of the tournament had taken its toll on his contact lenses, so they in turn had taken it out on his poor eyes.

At the very time in the game when Taylor needed his eyes and contact lenses to be at their best, they let him down. He gave up contact lenses for tournaments and thereafter used a variety of different glasses or often nothing at all. The solution to his problem came in the form of ultra-enlarged glasses (Figure 5.4). They look a little strange at first, but the optics are great for snooker. They are worn right up on the face, but when looking down the cue Taylor sees through the optically exact part of the lens – no more distortion. An added bonus is that the large, high glasses do not restrict the field of vision anywhere near as much as normal glasses.

Taylor started to wear the strange glasses in 1983 and stuck with them. At the 1984 World Championship he lost in the semifinals, but in 1985 he reached the final once again. He was up against Steve Davis, the greatest player of that time, who cruised into an eight frames to nil lead and his opponent looked as if he was sunk without trace. Taylor pulled himself back, however, and, in one of the classic finals of all time, he won on the last ball of the last frame. Many of us remember that match and the joy on Taylor's face as he raised his cue in victory. Perhaps, however, it would have been appropriate to have raised his glasses as well?

FACTS AND OLD WIVES' TALES

✧ It has often been said that Vincent Van Gogh (1853–90) must have had a visual problem to account for his vivid, personal style of painting. However, he had eye tests during his life and his vision was reported to be perfect.

✧ It has been suggested that John Constable (1776–1837) may have developed cataracts in later life, which could account for this painter's

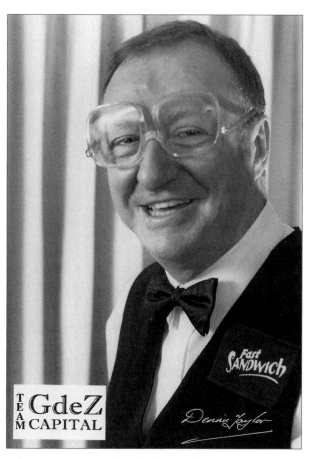

Figure 5.4 Dennis Taylor with his extra-large lenses extending high up onto his forehead.

preference for reds (see also Cézanne). Reds and browns do dominate his later works, but Constable hardly deserves Mark Twain's description of his paintings: 'like a ginger cat having a fit in a bowl of tomatoes'.

✧ The author and creator of Sherlock Holmes, Sir Arthur Conan Doyle (1859–1930), started his working life as a medical doctor in Southsea. He then became an eye specialist in London but made so little money at it that he turned to fiction writing to supplement his income.

Chapter 6

Eyes are us
Eyes and the way we live

In world mythologies the eye is frequently the emblem of light, power and wisdom – and often more than just wisdom, representing also the ability to read events in the future. Conversely, stupidity and ignorance are sometimes personified in the form of a blind god, or evil in the form of a sightless witch. It is not coincidental that some of the words we use for supernatural experiences are ocular. A seer has not necessarily got acute physical sight (often quite the opposite) and we understand 'a vision' as being quite separate from 'vision'. In religion the faithful 'see the light' and the sceptics are 'blind to the faith'.

In this chapter I will explore the power of the eye. This is not just the power of seeing; it goes beyond that. Eyes have a forceful influence on society through mythology, religious symbolism and philosophy. That we are a sight-dominated species influences everything from what we wear to what we build. However, our environment has changed to such an extent that our eyes are no longer protected to the degree they once were in the time of primitive man. Sight on the one hand is simply one of the five senses, but there is also the other hand …

MYTHICAL AND MYSTIC EYES

Research shows that way back in the neolithic period, in quite different parts of the world, an eye or a pair of eyes was the magic symbol that represented the goddess of fertility. These early cults may have had some influence on the mythology of ancient Egypt, where veneration of the eye reached an extraordinary level never quite matched anywhere else. A remnant of the Egyptian 'eye cult' survives on the back of a US dollar bill, which has an eye symbol on top of a pyramid.

Egypt

In Egyptian mythology the eye (all sorts of eyes) had a very special place,

138

so much so that saying their beliefs were eye-dominated may not be too strong. The eyes and their mysterious gift of sight must have had a profound influence on the day-to-day lives of the ancient Egyptian people because eye symbols became associated with the wonders and mysticism of their complex and ever-evolving religion. All they needed to do was look into the sky, day or night, and there was one of the eyes of their chief god. In Egyptian mythology one of the ancient beliefs was that the sun was the right eye of a great divine hawk while the moon was its left eye. The hawk god was the king of the gods and he went by several names as Egyptian religions developed and matured. He was Horus who had the head of a hawk and the body of a man, but he was also the sun god Ra, the creator.

Ra reigned in peace over people and gods until he became old, but when they knew he was no longer as strong and as powerful as he used to be, they plotted against him. When Ra found out that the people of the world no longer respected him, he became enraged and hurled down his eye to earth. The eye took the form of the goddess Hathor and killed many of his subjects, leaving only enough to ensure that mankind was not exterminated. When Ra had seen enough slaughter, he decided it was time to stop, but stopping Hathor was no easy business. While she was sleeping, Ra told his subjects to find all the best quality beer they could and mix it with some red ochre to look like blood. The avenging Hathor woke up the next day and set out on her path of destruction, only to find it blocked by a 'lovely' lake of blood. She drank and drank of this blood until she was quite tipsy, then forgot all about her mission and went merrily back home to be congratulated by Ra and turned back into the divine eye. Ra compromised with old age by dying at night, being reborn as a baby at dawn, growing to full manhood by midday and then declining once again.

Another story involves Ahnur, the god of battle, who is often depicted in ancient Egypt as a soldier wearing a headdress of feathers and carrying a strong spear. Ahnur left Egypt and went south into Nubia in search of the divine eye, which had gone missing. The warrior god eventually found the eye and brought it back to its home in Egypt. The divine eye was furious to find that, while it had been in Nubia, another eye had taken its place. Ra was pleased to have the divine eye home again and took it and placed it in the middle of his forehead. Here the divine eye became Uraeus whose job it was to protect the king of the gods from powerful enemies. It was also depicted in the form of a rearing but defensive cobra who watched over and protected the gods. The divine eye or *Iret eye* attained such a status that it could be considered to be a goddess in its own right.

There was a second Horus and that was the son of Osiris who was killed by his brother Seth. This Horus had the job of revenge on Seth, so, as you might imagine, the two of them quarrelled a good deal. During one of their many fights, Seth found Horus sleeping and tore out his left eye. The evil Seth ripped the eye to pieces and threw the remains beyond the edge of the world. The fragments were found by another god, called Thoth (the baboon god), who collected all of them and put them together again. The eye that Thoth put together is frequently associated with the moon and is known as the *Wedjat eye*. In the end Horus won the battle with Seth, so really the eye, in all its forms, won over darkness.

Egyptian mythology is dominated by the eye, or many eyes, but why is this a symbol of the great events such as day and night, the seasons, etc? In the words of R. T. Rundle Clark, an expert in Egyptology, 'The widespread popularity of the eye symbol must be based on common experience. Most peoples have been sensitive to the power and vitality which seem to reside in the eye. The Egyptians felt this so much that they exalted their feelings to cosmic dimensions.' The Egyptian family of mythical, often mystic, eyes were powerful and violent, often burning and terrible; given that ancient Egyptians (in common with their descendants today), through living in a very hot, dry and dusty climate, were prone to eye inflammations and worse, such as trachoma (see chapter 4), may there have been a medical and mythical association between the fiery, disturbing eyes of the cosmos and the troublesome ones of everyday life?

The various mystic and mythical eyes appear frequently in the hieroglyphic writings in numerous stylized forms. Sometimes, however, the eye symbols have a very practical worth. I once commented on a pair of eyes painted on an ancient Egyptian coffin in Liverpool Museum and asked what god was being symbolized. The reply was: 'They are for the mummy to look through into the after world.' It was refreshing after all the others to come across a very practical pair of eyes at last!

Babylon and Persia

A succession of powerful empires grew up in the fertile lands between the Tigris and Euphrates rivers, an early one being that of the Sumerians (about 3000 BC) and the last being that of the Babylonians (after 1800 BC). A rich culture went hand-in-hand with an imaginative mythology in which one of the great gods, Ea, was known as 'Lord of the Sacred Eye'. The eye in this case was one of knowledge and oracles, Ea being the god of supreme wisdom. He may have been a very clever god, but he was not a very attractive one and is often shown as having the body of a goat and the tail of a fish.

Much later Persian mythology had within it a ritual based on a drink of immortality called 'haoma', a fearsomely alcoholic brew fermented by a secret method from a sacred herb. The central figure was a god called Yimir the Splendid, with whom his followers could communicate after drinking haoma – and no doubt, after quaffing this they would have had very little ability to communicate with anyone else! Yimir was a deity of good and harmony who, through his possession of the solar eye, could make people and animals well, even 'non-mortal', prevent drought, sustain plants and crops, and protect people from evil spells. This was another example of a special eye with great power, although possibly not sufficient to save the followers from a haoma hangover!

Greece and Rome

Much of Roman mythology was imported from Greece with the result that although the names are different the stories are the same. Here I will use the Greek names with the Roman ones in brackets.

Strictly speaking, in this mythology there is not an 'eye god' as such, but Apollo (the same name to both Greeks and Romans), the sun god, is worth a mention in that context. He was the son of Zeus (Jupiter) and twin of Artemis (Diana), the goddess of hunting. Apollo, in both mythologies, is associated with light and was often referred to as the brilliant god. He was patron of archery and would rain down illnesses with his arrows; perversely he was also identified with healing and medicine. This Greco-Roman god comes close in his activities and status to the divine eye of the Egyptians.

Apollo was associated with Delphi because he slew the great serpent that lived there and then had to remain there himself for many years as a penance for his deed. Legend has it that the Delphic Oracle was founded by Apollo and here mythology merges with history. The ancient Greeks firmly believed that the temple at Delphi was the place to go to gain insight into the future. The priestess 'seer' would ramble, rave and spit a great deal, but out of this Apollo-inspired gibberish would come snippets of the future. The 'all-seeing eye' is common to many mythologies, including ancient Greek and Egyptian.

The cyclopes in Greek mythology are frightening because they are large man-eaters, but most of all because they have inhuman faces. A face with only a single eye positioned above the nose is a terrifying and very alien image. In Homer's *Odyssey*, his hero Odysseus (Ulysses) meets a cyclops who catches him and his crew and starts eating a few of them every evening; as they had killed off many of his goats, the cyclops may have felt justified in this. Odysseus and his men manage to blind the monster by ramming a stake into his one eye when he is drunk, and thereafter they make their escape. I wonder if the cyclops would have had more of our sympathy if he had had two eyes and looked more human?

Folklore, mythology and religion are full of tales about the glance of certain eyes having a devastating effect, as we have already appreciated with the eye of Horus (see also later the 'evil eye' and the 'third eye of Shiva').

There is also the forbidden glance – mythology is full of examples of people coming to a bad end because they have seen something they shouldn't have seen. The Greek goddess Athene (Minerva) was seen naked by Teiresias. Although the encounter was accidental, Athene had the poor man blinded, but as an afterthought gave Teiresias the gift of telling the future, which may have or may not have been some compensation. It was, however, preferable to the fate of the hunter Actaeon, who stumbled on Artemis (Diana) bathing in the nude. She turned him into a stag and he was set upon by his own hounds.

One of the best-known 'forbidden sight' stories is that of the Greek hero Perseus, and the gorgon, Medusa. Perseus embarked on a quest to find the Gorgon, but first he had to discover where she lived. He visited three old witches who shared one eye and one tooth between them. Perseus managed to steal the eye and the tooth, only returning them when he was told where the gorgon dwelt. Medusa had snakes for hair and was so ugly that anyone who looked at her was immediately turned to stone. Perseus overcame the problem by using the polished inside of his shield as a mirror. In this way he was able to get close to Medusa and cut off her head, which he placed in a bag. After many adventures, during which he turned kings and monsters to stone by taking out Medusa's head and showing it to them, he eventually gave the head to the goddess Athene who put it into the centre of her war shield.

Scandinavia and Germany

In Scandinavian and German mythology there is the sad story of Balder. Balder was a god of light and he was the best-loved son of Odin, the chief of the Nordic gods. Balder was a popular god because he was always happy and cheerful. However, there came a time when Balder was seen to be worried and withdrawn, quite out of character. The other gods asked what was wrong with him and Balder replied that he had had a series of bad dreams which foretold his death. His parents, Odin and Frigga, were very concerned about these dreams and Frigga in particular decided not to leave anything to chance. She visited every person and every thing and asked them to swear that they would never harm her son. This they did gladly, because they all liked Balder, so Frigga retired content that her precious son was safe.

The trouble with being popular is that there is always someone who is resentful of it, and in this case it was the evil god of fire, Loki. Loki was able to discover that one plant, the mistletoe, had been overlooked by Frigga and therefore was not bound by the oath of protection. Balder and his friends had a new game they enjoyed playing: they would throw sticks, stones, metal objects and all types of weapons at Balder but because of the oath they did him no harm. The evil Loki made a spear from mistletoe which he gave to Hother to throw at Balder. Hother was not a random choice: he was the blind god and brother to Balder. He did not join in the fun because he could not see. Loki said that he would help Hother and together they flung the spear at Balder, who was killed outright.

The gods tried all means to retrieve Balder from the underworld, but it was to no avail. Loki was caught and imprisoned in a magic net. Poor Hother, although he was blind and had been duped by Loki, did not avoid blame and retribution at the hands of Vali, the youngest son of Odin, who made it his duty to avenge the killing of the favourite god. Stories in mythology come uncomfortably close to equating blindness with stupidity or making blindness seem to be a fault rather than an affliction.

Some of the German/Saxon gods and also Celtic deities, in Britain and other parts of Europe, had a very bad press from the early Christians in the conflict of beliefs in which the eventual losers were the pagan deities. The horned gods conveniently became devils for the Christians to fear, while the moon goddesses of various sorts (and their followers) became witches. The moon goddesses had the cat as one of their chief symbols, mainly because cats' eyes dilate so dramatically at night to catch any rays of light there might be in the gloom, and in the day close down to narrow slits, thus reminding people of the waxing and waning of the moon (see Plate 7). The black cat was a particular favourite because all that can be seen at night are its big eyes glowing like the full moon. As a result the moon goddesses' symbol, the black cat, became the witches' 'familiar'.

The evil eye

The *evil eye* is an almost universally feared totem whereby a look can become a curse. An evil thought can be made effective by a particular look, and many different societies relate to the evil eye, creating myriad devices to ward off its effects. Christians, Muslims, Jews and Hindus all have a tradition that extends beyond their immediate and rational religious beliefs into superstition and, if not fear, then a fair degree of wariness. In various cultures a range of activities such as spitting, tattooing close to the mouth and eyes, wearing red, and carrying amulets (Plate 14), salt and even coal are thought to ward off the possible curse of the evil eye.

At Hogmanay in Scotland a piece of coal is handed to the host by the 'first footer', the first person across the threshold in the new year; at one level the coal is seen as a symbol of warmth, but at another it wards off the bad luck that might come from the evil eye. I once had a bookcase made for me by an excellent local carpenter. While it was being made, he asked if I might like to have a motif on the case and showed me some examples he had done in the past, which were superb. I thought for a while and then sent him a copy of the logo of my university department, which is in the form of an eye. When next I went into the carpenter's shop, he and his wife looked at me a little strangely until I explained that I worked in an eye department and was not wanting an evil eye symbol!

In the distant, and not too distant, past it was considered that 'rays' had to be emitted from the eye in order for the eye to be able to see. The idea that rays (of light) went into the eye and there was no two-way traffic was not accepted easily; such an eminent person as Euclid was a firm believer in the emanating rays theory. Nowadays, we still have some notion of rays coming out of the eye: consider Superman and his X-ray vision! The evil eye notion fits very comfortably with something coming from the eye, and thus the idea of visual emanations survives, even if it is now only associated with superheroes in comics and bad luck and malice in the 'real world'.

Mythology from elsewhere

There are many varied mythologies in the Pacific islands, but in several there is the belief that the sun and moon are eyes. In Mangaina (previously the Cook Islands), the sun and moon are the eyes of Vatea. Maoris of New Zealand also have a mythology in which the sun and moon are the eyes of heavenly creatures. The aborigines of New South Wales tell the story of the fight between the crane and the crow. It started when the crane one day had caught a load of fish and would not share them. The crow tried to steal some when the crane was distracted, but the crane turned round quickly and threw fish into the crow's eyes. The blinded crow fell into the fire and, when he finally escaped, his eyes had turned white from the fish and his feathers black from the flames.

Looking at the sun directly is a dangerous activity: as children some of us will have taken a magnifying lens and burnt paper by focusing the sun's rays. The cornea and, inside the eye, the lens are very good at focusing the sun's rays (see chapters 1 and 2), but instead of burning paper, sun-gazing means that the sensitive retina is fried and visual loss or blindness can be the consequence. West Indians, as with all people of the tropics, are wise to the dangers of the sun and in Jamaican and Caribbean lore there appears the character Anansi.

Anansi was the spider man, always up to no good, always in trouble, but always saved by his quick wits. His boasting was even too much for God, who called for Anansi to come up to heaven and sent him on an impossible quest 'for the night and the moon and the light of day'. The spider man returned, however, with a very big sack, put it down and reached in. The night he brought out of the sack turned heaven into pitch darkness. Next, out came the moon, and heaven was bathed in a silver glow. God was curious to see if Anansi had the sun, so he came closer thus getting the terrible brightness of the sun into his eyes. God cried out in pain and Anansi ran away, never to be seen again. When God looks down from heaven, there are small parts of the earth he can't see because of the sun burning in his eye. Smart people think that these parts are where you will find the spider man.

Mythology from around the world often tries to explain the differences between the sun and the moon, and I particularly like this myth from The Gambia. The sun and the moon were brother and sister, and on one occasion they went for a walk with their mother. The mother was hot, so she stopped by a waterfall and took off her clothes to have a cool bath in the waters. The sun was a good boy and turned his back so as not to embarrass his mother, but the moon had no such scruples and stared and stared at her mother's nakedness. After the bath their mother dressed and called the sun to her. She said how proud she was of him and she asked her god to grant that no one could look at him for any length of time. She was disgusted with her daughter, however, and wished of the moon that people could stare at her as long as they wanted.

EYE BELIEVE

I do not want to dwell on controversial aspects of comparative religion, except to make the point that sight is an important facet of our belief, no matter what that belief may be. However, the danger of my over-simplification of complex matters is all too apparent.

Christianity

John Hull, a professor of religious education at Birmingham University, went blind when he was 40 years of age. He became dismayed by the imagery of the Bible which equates light with good and darkness with evil. To him it was self-evident that the Bible was written by sighted people, for sighted people, but even knowing that does not provide much comfort for the visually handicapped when blindness is presented almost as a sin.

I had not thought of the Bible in quite this way, but once it was pointed out, realized it is true that imagery of 'lightness' on one hand and 'darkness' on the other is to the forefront of the whole story of Jesus. Scanning quickly through the Gospels of the New Testament, it is easy to find eye and vision references.

An example is the opening verses of St John, about John the Baptist, which are full of light references. Chapter 1, verses 4 and 5 say: 'In him was life; and the life was the light of men. And the light shineth in darkness; and the darkness comprehended it not.' Later, verses 8 and 9 state, about John: 'He was not that Light, but was sent to bear witness of that Light.

That was the true light that lighteth every man that cometh into the world.' These verses create very powerful images, going further than equating light with goodness and faith, and saying that the 'Light' is Jesus himself. There are, of course, many more of these references in the New Testament, so that Christians are used to considering God as the 'Light' and Jesus as the 'Light of the World'.

Direct mention of eyes, vision in both senses of the word, blindness and so forth are to be found throughout the Gospels and the whole of the New Testament. An appropriate example would be the famous eye reference from St Mark, which runs: 'And if thine eye offend thee, pluck it out: it is better for thee to enter the Kingdom of God with one eye, than having two eyes to be cast into hell fire' (chapter 9, verse 47).

John Hull, the Birmingham University professor, was absolutely right with his observations on the Bible, but perhaps understandably over-sensitive about the meaning of the Word of God. For the Gospel writers trying to get their message across to the people of the Middle East and elsewhere, equating light with good and dark with bad is powerful imagery that had also been used to great effect in the Old Testament (see Judaism). In addition, loss of eyesight would have been an all too common affliction in the hot, sandy and insanitary conditions of the Holy Land two thousand years ago (see chapter 4, e.g. trachoma). The consequence of blindness to those people must have been a dire and readily understood horror.

Islam

It is believed by many Muslims that certain looks convey curses that bring bad luck to the victim. Such beliefs are a part of Islamic culture, although not part of the actual religious faith as far as I am aware. Amulets to ward off the effects of such looks abound in the Middle East. One amulet, known as the 'Hand of Fatima', is stylized to avoid the sin of creating a graven image, which is contrary to all Islamic faith, and is thought to provide the hand of protection to those who carry it. A further bonus is to have on the amulet a pair of eye devices, which returns the curse back to the person who sent it in the first place!

Judaism

At the very start of the Old Testament in Genesis the opening words are: 'In the beginning God said "let there be light" and there was light.' Light comes before the universe in order of priority for mankind, emphasizing in the most important of Jewish and, for that matter, Christian books the significance of sight and the repugnance of profound blackness. The overriding importance of sight could not have been stressed any more than it is. The imagery is as evident in the Old Testament as it is in the New (see

Christianity). I suspect that the emphasis on 'seeing and not seeing' and 'light and dark' should be placed in the context of a desert people in the Middle East with limited resources. The day would be harsh but glorious, whereas the night would be cold and inhospitable.

Again straying away from religion, there is a common belief, deep set in the culture of Jews in various parts of the world, that eye symbols are protective and ward off evil. To this end, girls have bracelets of multiple eye symbols and adult women wear necklaces with amulets of stylized eyes incorporated into the design.

Hinduism

Shiva is one of the more important Hindu gods, and is frequently known as 'the destroyer'. He is usually pictured with an ashen white face and a blue neck gained from swallowing poison at the world's beginning. He has a number of associated objects or symbols which include a garland of snakes, a string of skulls, the crescent moon and, of particular significance, a third eye.

The awesome power of this extra eye has the ability to reduce the world to a cinder if so required and according to Hindu legend it burnt the god Kama to a crisp. The belief that there is an invisible third eye above the nose is reinforced in Indian culture by caste marks sited there and also possibly the 'tilaka' marking worn by Hindu wives.

Buddhism

The third eye was not always a terrible weapon as it seems to have been in Egyptian mythology and for the Hindu god Shiva. In Buddhism, a third eye denotes wisdom and spirituality. Some sculptures and paintings of Buddha show a very prominent third eye, which is an indication of the fact that he is on the way to heavenly bliss. However, even Buddhism doesn't avoid the vengeful additional eye entirely because it is prominent in a range of ferocious deities; there are, for example, two manifestations in Japanese Buddhism that have an extra eye, and another one with three extra eyes. One of these Buddhas has four heads, each with the additional eye in the forehead; another has only one head but makes up for it by sporting five distinctive eyes. The final one has an awful face with the three glaring eyes and a mouthful of fangs; a human skull acts as a hat. Despite the obvious problems with the face, this divinity is popular because it supports the poor and needy.

SOCIAL(EYES)

We are a species which visualizes and everything we are is visual; we see through our eyes and brain, but we think in pictures. If you shut your eyes and have no visual input, images will still course through your head like a disjointed movie. We cannot escape; a blind person has no eyesight but still thinks in pictures.

Mother's eye

The eye of a newborn baby is small and the density of cones is not great. From then on, the eye grows rapidly so that when the baby is six months of age, the eye is about 50 per cent larger than at birth. Subsequently growth slows down, and by six or seven years the eye has reached more or less its maximum size, and the density of cones, particularly in the central region, is also fully established. The baby's little eye is long-sighted and generates fuzzy, poorly focused vision. Despite limited vision in the first few months of life, however, the baby can recognize a face, although it will just be a blur. The baby goes from recognizing a face as an important pattern to being able to distinguish one face from another. The eyes of a three-month-old baby have some colour vision and are constantly moving and picking up visual information about its environment. The baby can even follow moving objects of interest, although not very smoothly. This is when mum, dad and the mobile above the cot are the most important things in the baby's life.

It is known that from a period before two months of age, when vision is still very fuzzy, the baby and its mum have developed a rapport that is surprisingly advanced (surprising only to scientists, never to mums and dads). The baby and parent communicate information to each other in many different ways: sound, touch, movement and of course sight. The baby's relatively poor vision is no handicap to the two-way exchange; in fact, it may be an advantage since peripheral images are not seen and are therefore no distraction. The interchange of facial expression, reactive response, mimicking and so on is so rich that psychologists call it *proto-conversation*.

Eye-to-face and even eye-to-eye contacts become well established at this stage in life as an important part of the communication process. From four months onwards the baby has more co-ordination and more strength, and becomes more involved with objects round about. Throughout early life, learning and play require reassurance, reward and encouragement. The emotional and physical dependence that a child has on its parents involves sight as an influential but not essential part of early social development.

Contacting eyes

Human beings make rather elaborate gestures with their hands and bodies (in some countries more than others) as part of conversation and communi-cation. In addition there is a whole repertoire of much more subtle movements that contribute to conversation and expression, which collectively can be called body language. The eyes rather than the ears are the receiver for much of this type of communication. If you really want to know what a friend is feeling, would you find out more easily from a phone conversation or from one held face-to-face, even if you used the same words for both?

People often say that someone has 'expressive eyes', and Shakespeare wrote of one of his characters, 'There's language in her eye.' This is not too far from the truth. As well as being the receivers for body language, the eyes are the masters of this type of communication. They are considered to give out a stream of messages, recognized almost at the subconscious level by the observer. These may consist of little more than a slight change in eye position, a minuscule dilation of the pupil or a twitch of an eyelid, but they provide a deep if not rich language of their own. People's interpretation of this type of language develops in the community, but is given a kick-start in those early days of infancy when they look into their mother's eyes.

There is constant reference to eye language in everyday writing and speech. We may be familiar with novels or magazine stories that describe how the young heroine 'fluttered her eyelashes with embarrassment' or how the hero is 'full of resolve with eyes of flint'. We can recall conversations such as 'He didn't say so to my face, but I know he was the guilty one; his eyes gave him away,' or 'Jane was just as frightened as I was when we realized there was a bull in that field. Her eyes went as big as saucers and there was a definite twitch in one of them!'

Our eyes are hostage to our emotions, or more accurately to our body chemistry of hormones and the like. We have learned to read the subtle changes in response to emotion, for example, the pupils widen and the lids go back a little when we are frightened or excited: 'eyes as big as saucers'. This comment illustrates how well tuned in we are to this type of signalling; the pupil widens only marginally and the lids open just a trifle, but describing the eyes as 'as big as saucers' is not considered absurd.

A slight widening of the pupils also occurs when we meet someone we like, so it is not surprising therefore that, when people are given a selection of pictures of faces, there is a general preference for those with wide pupils (in Figure 1.1 in chapter 1, the model has dilated pupils – probably she is responding to the excitement of the fashion show). The social importance of eyes as suppliers of information and signals is perhaps the reason for the persistence in many societies of the myth about emanations or rays coming from the eyes.

Certain minor taboos (good manners) have developed about how the eyes are held in conversation. In western countries some level of eye contact is taken to be a sign of openness when meeting someone, otherwise it might be said, for example, that 'He was shifty, he wouldn't look me straight in the eye!' In other societies, such as those of Japan, India and the Middle East, avoidance of eye contact can be good manners, while eye contact may be considered disrespectful (employee to employer) or brazen (woman to man). In the past, fans, which on one level have a cooling action in stuffy conditions, on another were used by ladies to hide their facial and eye gestures. With the fan as a mask, it was difficult to read the facial language, but the action of the fan itself often became a substitute.

It seems to be an unwritten rule of contact that, even in societies where sporadic eye contact is seen to be a good thing, the amount of eye contact rapidly diminishes the closer in proximity two people are to each other (the exception is, of course, if the two people are in a close relationship). To see an example of the extreme avoidance of eye contact that occurs when strangers get too close to each other, take a trip on the London Underground during rush hour. It is amazing how so many people manage to look at absolutely nothing all at the same time.

Forcing yourself to have little or no eye movement is an extreme type of eye-to-eye signal which is meant to be intimidating. Two boxers in the ring at the beginning of a fight often indulge in staring each other out, and this is certainly frightening to the audience if not to them. Parents, schoolteachers and lecturers may develop their own 'withering stare' to convey to children and students that they are not pleased.

Attraction between the sexes is an extremely complex biological and social process, but sight plays much more than a minor role. On the basis of social surveys, it has been found that physical appearance is a major factor in attraction, although the appearance of the female is more important for the male than vice versa. Studies that investigate what a subject is looking at when looking at another person all come up with the same thing: our eyes come to rest far more often on the face than any other part of the body, and within the face it seems to be the eyes that attract the majority of the attention. Consequently it would seem that in the game of attraction, as in social communication, 'the eyes have it'.

Dreamy eyes

Dreaming, unlike seeing, does not involve immediate input from the eyes, but as human beings dream in pictures it is valid to mention it. The mechanics of dreaming are not well understood, but the ability to dream seems to be housed in the *cerebral cortex* of the brain; if this is damaged, the individual sleeps a great deal but never dreams. The pattern of normal sleep for most people reaches a very deep level at first, then climbs to much lighter sleep, and then down again, and so on. During an eight-hour sleep period, there would be about five lighter sleep levels, taking up roughly an hour and a half of the total. The lighter sleep periods are associated with considerable brain activity and strange movement of the eyes. The eyelids are closed, but beneath them the eyeballs dart rapidly backwards and forwards. This is termed *rapid eye movement* (REM).

People usually wake up soon after their last REM phase and most dreams that are remembered will have occurred during this period. Often dreams appear to have filled the whole night, but in reality they take up very little time. People who say they don't dream are always shown to be as active as anyone else when they are fitted to brain-wave recording instruments; they just do not remember their dreams. Dreaming is like having your own picture show, but one where the images and dialogue often don't make much sense when recalled, even when they seemed to make perfect sense when you were experiencing them.

What do dreams mean? The psychoanalysts from Sigmund Freud onwards think they have some of the answers but, unfortunately, they disagree profoundly among themselves. There is a belief that dream images are symbols and can be interpreted like a language. I have no idea whether this is true, but the bookshop and library shelves have plenty of books on how to interpret dreams, and I am as guilty as the next person of picking them up and browsing through. These books are amazing, if only because they illustrate the huge range of things human beings dream about.

Moral (eyes)

Much of this chapter, and for that matter much of this book, has been concerned with the special place of eyes. There is the tangible role of our eyes as the dominant sense organ, but there is also the less tangible role, an almost mystical capacity, which is summed up in the metaphor that the eye is the window of the soul. The association of the eyes with philosophy and inner wisdom runs through many, if not all, societies and past civilizations. For that matter, the frequent references to the eye in various mythologies probably were attempts to personify, among other things, the mystic role of the inner eye.

I do not intend to dwell very long on the metaphysical aspects of the eye, but a very appropriate quote to keep in mind comes from Lord Bowden (1835–94), who described a person who deals with *metaphysics* as 'A blind man in a dark room looking for a black hat which isn't there.' Nonetheless, the link between the eyes, morality and the soul has had, and still has, too strong a hold in our societies just to be dismissed out of hand.

There is a deep-rooted feeling that, if there is any gateway to the soul, then it is through the eyes, a notion captured by the poet Ezra Pound (1885–1972): 'To have gathered from the air a live tradition or from a fine old eye the unconquered flame'. The belief that the inner self shines through the eyes may well contribute to the importance of the eye as something more than just an important sense organ. The link between the eye and the soul is such that one of the first things done after death is to close the lids. For that matter, in days gone by it was traditional to place pennies on the eyes of a corpse (an old penny was large enough more or less to cover the eye). In some ways lifeless eyes seem to be more disturbing than a lifeless body.

Eye impact

It is difficult to grasp just how much of what human beings are and what they have become is due to the fact that they are dexterous, social animals gifted with large brains and good eyesight. It does mean that what we make does not always need to be functional, but even when it is functional it often needs to be appealing. Good or bad taste has nothing to do with the mouth, but plenty to do with the impact on the eye. Our vision is so dominant that it is hard to think of an aspect of our society that is not influenced to a lesser or greater extent by the fact that we are a species ruled by our sight. However, I will start with something very close to us: clothes.

Clothes are functional necessities that protect us from the heat of the sun, the beating rain, the howling wind and the freezing snow. With shoes or boots on our feet, we can tackle rugged or muddy terrains with equal disdain. Hats of various types keep out the rain, bring warmth in the cold and give shade when it is hot. Human beings are the furless species that can produce its own coverings in a bewildering range of materials and forms, which far extends the range of climates in which we can live and has allowed us to populate the world at large.

We all know that clothes have an extremely important practical function, but that is not the end of it. Clothes are also worn to make a visual statement in our society, along with jewellery, hair styling, tattoos, make-up (see later section on this) and other accessories. After all, a western woman does not go out wearing an expensive necklace because of the need to carry her wealth with her, nor does a man with a Rolex watch have a desperate need to know the time. Fashion has little or nothing to do with functional necessity and everything to do with 'looking nice' and being admired. Smart clothes make us feel good and say something about us to other people. They extend sexuality, although one of their supposed roles is to dampen down sex signals. I must admit to being sceptical about the latter, because one of the most sexless places I can think of from a signalling point of view is a nudist colony!

If humans were not a visually orientated species, the fashion industry would not exist and neither would the amazing variety of clothes we wear. My mother has four or five wardrobes full of clothes and surprisingly she wears most of them at one time or another. Other people have more modest numbers of clothes, but that is more often than not because they throw some away soon after they buy something new. How often have you thrown clothes out because they are worn out, and how often because you 'wouldn't want to be seen dead in that'? This would not happen if we were a purely functional species that was not so heavily visually orientated.

Clothes are a signalling device that says such things as: 'I am rich and can afford to wear designer labels'; 'I am an attractive woman and can get away with wearing sexy things'; 'I am a football supporter and wear my team's colours'; 'I am a rebel and do not wish to conform'; and so on. From the following description, can you tell anything about the person? 'Wears a Saville Row two-piece pin-striped suit and the trousers have a sharp crease. Jewellery includes a Cartier gold watch and a thick gold ring on the third finger of the left hand. A flower in the buttonhole, an immaculate white shirt, silk tie and shiny black hand-made leather shoes set it all off.' A reasonable guess could be made at the person's sex, age range, type of work, marital status, habits and, speculatively, at their standing in the community. All this and more can be gleaned from the previous description yet that description is restricted to what the person is wearing.

This does not stop at clothes, of course. Our homes are an extension of our 'taste', and much of that is about what we find visually pleasing and to a certain extent what we think other people will also find visually pleasing. We need curtains for privacy and carpets for warmth, but they don't have to be fancy to be functional, do they? Why have pictures on the wall and what earthly good are ornaments on the ledges or in a glass case? The outside of the house has visual features as well: the garden with its well-cut lawn and colourful flowers, for instance. A garden, or its equivalent, at one time had the functional role of providing food to eat. For the most part, we still have a garden because it pleases us and gives us the right visual signals, but as a practical proposition it is a waste of time. For example, to take the argument to the extreme, the Palace at Versailles, the Summer Palace at St Petersburg and Hampton Court Palace are only places built for people to live in, and their gardens were never constructed to provide food for any table!

Visual order pleases many (although not all) of us, and this extends to the town and country parks that are an extension of our personal gardens on a communal scale. If these were just places for children to run and for walking dogs, there would be no need for all the rich and colourful banks of flowers or the 'keep off the grass' signs. Psychologists have shown that large parkland areas (Richmond Park, Windsor Great Park, etc.) with broad tracts of green grass, small clumps of trees or high bushes and some water represent our most relaxing and preferred environment. It is also close to the savannah type of country where we developed as a species, and ideal for a relatively slow, cunning primate with excellent eyesight to survive and thrive.

In a small heavily populated country such as Britain, much of the countryside has been tamed and altered by the farmers and people who live there. The layout, order and geometry of the countryside can best be appreciated from the air, and can be seen to be dictated to some extent by the economic fact that the design is efficient for sight-dominated people to herd enclosed animals and take in crops.

We do not build our churches, institutional and commercial buildings, and sometimes even our factories, in a strictly utilitarian manner. The design, the fabric, and in fact the whole structure with any embellishments make visual statements that produce an emotional response in those who see them, which may be indifference, wonder, pride, horror, outrage, etc. If we were not a visually orientated species, we would not, for example, be investing heavily in a new British Library in London. We would not have books in the first place, and arguments about whether the appearance of the new building is more attractive than the old would be pretty fatuous.

As well as the libraries of the world, great and small, all the many art galleries, museums and monuments would be a waste of time and space were it not for our visual nature. Most monuments and statues only make visual sense; after all, would a sightless species or even a species with poor vision bother having, for example, the Eiffel Tower (Figure 6.1), Trafalgar Square, the Statue of Liberty, etc? The question is rhetorical: they all bring pleasure, pride, wonder and a number of other emotions to the soul through the eyes.

Places of worship can be extremely simple; a wooden shack may be all that one group of Christians requires, although another group has the lavish trappings of a baroque cathedral. Religious wars and schisms have had, as one of their causes, a disagreement about the adornment of churches. On the one hand it is held that a beautiful and lavishly adorned church is a tribute to God, and on the other that such extravagance is sinful. It could be argued that both are the responses of a sight-dominated people to their religion, because both extremes of church style make a visual statement. Ornate churches are built as shrines to the glory of God (or perhaps to the ingenuity and wealth of man), but the very understatement of the simplest church gives out an equally powerful statement regarding the notion that austerity is next to godliness. In impact of visual message, there is little to choose between the two.

Advert(eyes)

The image is all-powerful in our lives, and sight is the sense we most trust, which is borne out by the saying 'seeing is believing'. The evidence of our other senses usually needs to be double checked before we are satisfied, and

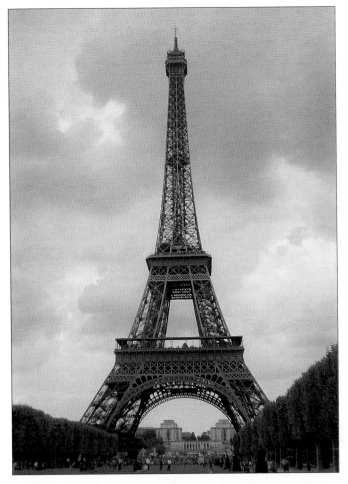

Figure 6.1 The Eiffel Tower: only a sight-dominated species would ever have built it.

more often than not it is sight that provides the assurance: 'Go and see if the toast is all right in the kitchen, I think I can smell burning'; 'I think I heard a noise downstairs; I'll just get up and see what it is'; and 'I've picked up something at the back of the cupboard that feels so bad I daren't look at it!'

We are quite sceptical about the spoken word, and less so about the written word, but we find it difficult not to believe what is in a picture – a picture 'never lies'. Pictorial images are powerful persuaders, whether they be photographs, films, television or the Internet, so much so that they can blur the edges between reality and fantasy. Many of us have tears running down our cheeks when a film has a sad ending, because we have been emotionally involved with the story. Yet we still know on another level that the film is not real, and it is the product of the collective efforts of actors, writers, directors, etc.

Television and films merely exploit, and are substitutes for, the capacity we have for creating scenes in our head. Imagination has survival value for our species by allowing us to think ahead and to plan for a host of eventualities. The moving image, in whatever form, is merely a descendant of a cultural tradition that goes back to the fireside storyteller and has carried on from the written book and the acted play. All require us to make a step from reality to fantasy; this is as true for the non-fictional documentary type of report as it is for any make-believe story.

After all, we don't have a jungle, a football stadium, a down-town street, a prison or whatever in our living room, but our television will take us there. It will involve us in a famine, a riot, a disaster or even a war, and the way in which the images are presented to us has the capacity to influence our emotions and our opinions, the subject at hand. The images we see are, hopefully, balanced in presentation, but this is not always the case. It may be a very obvious thing to say, but television or film news, views and documentaries are as edited and selected as in any newspaper. I'm not saying this is either good or bad, just that these media are not reality, which we accept on the level of reason but find far harder to grasp emotionally. The healthy scepticism we have for most forms of persuasion seems to be less robust when faced with a picture, moving or otherwise.

Our susceptibility to pictorial evidence is exploited nowhere more bla-tantly than in advertising. Advertising attempts to influence our behaviour by an assault on our senses, particularly our eyes. The old adage that a picture is worth a thousand words is the war cry of the advertising agency (Plate 15). To work well, the advertising image has to have sufficient impact for us to want to look at it, an easy up-front message and probably a more subtle message not entirely obvious to our conscious mind but which works away at our subconscious.

Vance Packard called the advertisers who appeal at these two different levels *The Hidden Persuaders* in the 1950s, and the message of his book about the subtleties of advertising technique are still valid today (an edition was published in the 1990s – see Further Reading). As I understand it, the subconscious messages appeal to our greed, our fears, our need to be liked, our sex drive, and so on. It is no coincidence that in an advert for a car a smart young man is driving it in an exotic location with a stunning young woman at his side. Not only is the car being sold; the advert is also selling an image of how you might like to be and telling you that buying the car is a key to that fantasy lifestyle. The box of chocolates is not sold just on the basis that such things are nice to eat, but that they are eaten exclusively by the rich, the bold and the beautiful.

See at sea

Becoming lost at sea can have fatal consequences now, but in the days before the radar or even the compass, it was a sailor's great fear. Portuguese fishing boats and Asian junks of various types often had a pair of bright eyes painted on the prow to show them where to go, or at least to impart confidence that the boat was looking out at the way ahead, giving the crew good luck or perhaps just looking for a shoal of fish. Even the great Viking seamen, with their beautiful dragon-headed longships, made sure that the carved dragon had a big pair of eyes looking to the front. Men-of-war had distinctive carved figureheads which were there first of all to bring the ship good fortune, but also to help the ship see through fog banks or bad weather. Of course, large eyes at the front of a ship of war must have been quite frightening when they were seen coming towards you; Chinese fighting junks used eye motifs to great effect.

BEAUTIFUL EYES

Charles Darwin in his *Origin of Species* put forward his theories on natural selection and evolution. Outlined in the book are many of the 'fors' and some of the 'againsts' with regard to evolution, but one thing that gave him considerable problems was the eye. How could a simple process of selection culminate in something as complex and intricate as the human eye or the eye of an eagle, in Darwin's words 'organs of extreme perfection and complication'? The answer would seem to be that, given enough time, anything is possible, but in society we try to make 'extreme perfection' even better through the use of make-up.

Past eyes

Eye make-up was common in many cultures in the past as it is in cultures today. The original use of eye make-up was in most cases not intended to beautify the eyes but to act as a defence mechanism. The defence was either spiritual or, less commonly, medical. Dyes and various substances, sometimes in conjunction with tattooing and appropriate jewellery, were plastered around the eyes, sometimes in intricate patterns, to protect them from the invasion of evil spirits and such like.

Many societies in diverse parts of the world at different times took such precautions very seriously indeed. They held that evil spirits or genii made entry into the body through its openings and these needed to be guarded appropriately. The main opening you might have thought would be the mouth, but it does seem that the eyes were considered to be a particularly vulnerable gateway. Perhaps because it is believed in many societies that the 'eyes are the windows to the soul', they need to be surrounded by charms that drive the spirits away.

Remnants of these traditions still exist in the world today or have died out in the recent past. Children in many parts of India still have their eyes and cheeks blackened with lamp soot to make them a less obvious target for spirits. In parts of North Africa, a silver headband worn by the women has an extension that drops between the eyes on to the top of the nose; this and other adornments keep at bay evil influences including the evil eye. Berber women wear the silver nose drop, but some also have beneath their eyes rows of coloured dots which can be green, red or white.

The Berbers are not unique. There are a number of African, Asian and South American societies where white metal, usually silver or alloy, is used to protect vulnerable parts from the invasion by evil spirits. The metal that guards the 'openings' is often in the form of rings or studs. There is currently an enthusiasm for body piercing with surgical steel rings (lips, tongue, nose and eyebrows) among the young and the young at heart in the West. I wonder if they know that their fashion statement arose in other cultures because of a fear of spiritual invasion?

For the origins of eye make-up, beginning with its medicinal role, we return to ancient Egypt once again. The people were quite health conscious and they had a definite concern for their eyes (see chapter 3), which is not surprising given the prominence of eyes in their religious beliefs. They indulged in 'preventive medicine' on a grand scale and rubbed a black mixture called *kohl* around their eyes.

Kohl started life as a medical paste but, because it became more and more important in Egyptian society, it evolved into a cosmetic. This was the eye make-up of all eye make-ups; kohl was so important to Egyptian society that it had to be applied each day to the lids and brows, and no respectable Egyptian male or female would be seen without it – rather like seventeenth-century Europeans and their wigs. Even statues had to have their daily eye make-over; nothing escaped without having kohl around his, her or its eyes.

Eye make-up became more sophisticated and elaborate, especially for women. Much care and attention was needed, plus a steady hand, so a special wooden arm-rest was developed. Kohl was painted on as a thick black line through the eye brows and as a thinner line around the eye; inside this black ring, a green powder made from malachite was applied to the upper and lower lids to make the eyes stand out. Cleopatra had her own exclusive pattern of eye make-up, which was basically to colour the upper lid dark blue and the lower one green. Surprisingly kohl is still used today by a few Arab children who have it rubbed on their upper and lower lids by their parents. It started as a medicine, became a cosmetic and now is used to ward off the effects of the 'evil eye' – the complete circle.

Western eyes

Eye make-up is hugely important in western society as part of a woman's visual appearance (Plate 16) and a quick glance in a beauty magazine will show how involved eye enhancement is. Eye make-up, I am told, is designed to make the eyes stand out because we consider that people with 'big' eyes are attractive. Big eyes are also a sign of openness and honesty, someone to trust. On the other hand, small deep-set eyes, particularly if the eyebrows are thick and meet over the nose, are considered to be full of menace. Big eyes well separated are 'good'; small eyes close together definitely are not 'good'. Marilyn Monroe, Frank Sinatra ('old blue eyes'), ET, Elizabeth Taylor and Mel Gibson are individuals deemed to have the former, along with bush babies (primitive monkeys with huge eyes).

In the beauty salon and at home, women's eyes are made more prominent by reducing the eyebrows by plucking to thin lines that definitely do not meet up. The lids are coloured to give them fullness and to contrast or tone with eye colour. Eyelashes are lengthened and thickened with mascara – the longer and thicker the better, because long lashes help to attract attention to the eyes and make them stand out. A pencil line behind the lashes adds to the overall effect. If mascara doesn't make the lashes sufficiently long and thick, then there are always false eyelashes to fall back on. Cosmetic contact lenses are fashionable in some quarters to give more striking eye colour; some companies even produce patterned lenses.

The skin beneath the brow and on the lid is dusted with coloured powder, again to highlight the eyes by introducing contrast. An additional benefit is to hide any wrinkles there may or may not be. Eye-to-eye contact is such an important factor in social communication in many societies that ever so slight imperfections around the eyes are often a cause of some distress. The small wrinkles that come with ageing, and are so harmless in themselves, can cause so much concern to both women and men alike.

Eastern eyes

Eye make-up is important in non-western cultures, but the context and the message given out might be quite different. In India the dot painted on the forehead of women, above the nose, indicates their marital status, but its origins are as an eye symbol. Followers of the god Shiva paint three white parallel lines on their forehead and in the middle is a prominent red dot which is a symbol for Shiva's third eye of knowledge.

EYELIGHTS

Research and development in modern society has produced a bewildering number of visual aids, which we mostly take for granted, but they are awesome. Modern society and the way we live, on the other hand, may be making demands on our eyes with which they were never designed to cope. The eye is the ultimate light receptor, but it is ironic that the very thing it was designed to capture and use, light, is also damaging to the delicate structure of the eye.

Eye see

Human eyes see more than any eyes have ever done. This is not because they are the best eyes in the animal kingdom. Rather it is because humans live in a highly visually orientated society and a considerable amount of their creative drive has been directed towards enhancing and extending what can be seen.

Inventive ingenuity has led to the development of the light microscope, which allows us to see individual cells and even germs such as bacteria. The electron microscope takes us even further on the journey of magnification, so that viruses and even the molecules of life can be appreciated. The magnifying glass has also evolved into the telescope with which we can see the planets and the stars. The most sophisticated radio telescopes can enhance our vision beyond our own stars to those of more distant galaxies. Visual information can be generated by means of modern telescopes from bodies so far away that the light from them started its journey across the vast reaches of space millennia before Christ was born.

Cameras allow us to record single images for posterity, a fleeting view captured in time. Digital technology now lets us transfer these images into the computer to modify or evaluate them. The cine-camera and its successor the video-camera can capture both image and movement in time. They are used to entertain us, but they are also part of the fabric of our life and exploration. The high-speed camera takes many shots in the blink of an eye so that even the passage of a bullet or the disintegration of a rain drop as it hits the ground can be studied and analysed frame by frame. The time-lapse camera is used to record events that occur over a prolonged period for replaying in as short a time as is comfortable. What takes hours, for example, the opening of a flower, can be seen in seconds, and what takes days, for example, the incubation and hatching of birds' eggs, can be seen in minutes. The time-lapse system of the scientist is now the security camera of most malls, businesses, banks, shops and supermarkets.

Combined with fibre-optic light guides and special lenses, the camera, video and television give us the ability to venture far and wide. Television and appropriate probes allow us to explore the depths of the sea where the pressure is so high we would be crushed to death in an instant. With such instruments we can examine the inside of active volcanoes, where we would be burnt to a crisp. We venture into environments that are poisonous (the inside of a chemical tank), dangerous (remote bomb disposal machines rely on a video link), risky (getting to the middle of a termite nest or an alligator swamp by camera is much more comfortable than doing it in person) or unpleasant (a journey into a sewer by video or a journey to an ulcer with an endoscope spring to mind).

I wonder which of these marvels would most impress our ancestors? I suspect it might be something that I have not mentioned so far, something we completely take for granted. I suspect that high on their list of marvels would be the creation of the 24-hour day by lighting up our homes, shops, places of entertainment, factories, streets and motorways. Some scientists have concerns about the effect that this and several of our other modern marvels have, or with time are going to have, on Charles Darwin's 'organs of extreme perfection' – our eyes!

Eye don't

Our ancestors first lived among the gentle greens and browns of the forest canopy. Good acuity helped to pick out bright berries and fruit to eat, but also was essential for the hand-to-eye co-ordination needed to swing through trees. The aerial acrobatics of present-day gibbons give us some idea of what was needed. At some point our ancestors left the trees and lived on the savannah lands, the plains of Africa. Early humans thrived in this environment, but it was not necessarily ideal for their eyesight. Heavy brow ridges, a mobile pupil, blinking and a downward gaze would have helped to provide protection. On the cynical side, however, the relatively short life of a hunter-gatherer would also have ensured that the eyes of early humans were in reasonably good shape throughout their life.

Society up until relatively recently lived by the clock; torch- and candle-light could stimulate rod vision, but little in the way of cone vision. Starlight and moonlight barely help a species with a cone-dominant retina, so travelling the rutted roads of yesteryear by night can't have been pleasant. Humans tried to conquer the night with oil lamps in the eighteenth century and gaslight in the nineteenth, but never truly succeeded until the latter half of the twentieth century when universal electric and neon lighting took over in the richest countries. Las Vegas stands in the middle of the Nevada Desert, which, like most deserts, is profoundly black at night. As you approach the city plane or car, you first become aware of an eerie glow on the horizon. As you get closer, the canopy of stars is blotted out as the glow gets brighter and brighter, and you can make out many colours and hues. If you travel towards Las Vegas at night in a small aircraft it is quite spooky: a dome of light extends high into the sky and beyond the city limits in all directions. Welcome to the city that never sleeps! I think that Las Vegas is the twentieth century's monument to the arrival of the 24-hour day.

I have hinted that our modern lighting and other facets of our society and way of life may contribute to the deterioration of vision. This is a most controversial area, but there is now quite a list of scientists who have linked environmental factors to the increased prevalence of some of the more common age-related eye diseases. What is beyond doubt is that more and more people are living longer lives, so greater numbers will contract age-related eye disease (see chapters 4 and 7) and many are in danger of out-living useful eyesight (see chapters 5 and 7).

Light is made up of different wavelengths, some of which we see and these wavelengths fall in what is called the visible range. There are others that we do not see. Outside the visual spectrum the short wavelengths fall in the ultraviolet range, while the long wavelengths are in the infra-red. As mentioned in chapter 2, certain animals, for example bees, can see into the ultraviolet. In turn, the ultraviolet and infra-red are subdivided, into UV-A, UV-B and UV-C for ultraviolet (each one of progressively shorter wavelength), A, B and C for infra-red, with the longest wavelength being C.

All light, visible or otherwise, is damaging to our eyes but some wavelengths are more problematic than others. The ultraviolets and the far infra-reds do not penetrate far into the eye when exposure occurs, because they are absorbed mostly by the outer coats of the eye. The last barrier to their penetration is the lens. On exposure to the long wavelengths of far infra-red, skin will fry and so will cornea, and such wavelengths will also produce a thermal (heat-related) cataract in the lens itself. The far ultraviolet, UV-C, also causes the cornea to become opaque and badly inflamed through photochemical (light-based) reactions in the tissue. The near ultraviolet, UV-A, is mostly absorbed in the lens where it can produce a cataract, while UV-B has the ability to produce both corneal opacity and cataract. Finally, near infra-red passes through deep into the eye where it is absorbed by the retina. It can burn the lens causing a cataract, and also the retina, bringing visual loss.

These extremes of high and low wavelengths are present in sunlight, but also in equipment used at home and at work. UV-A is part, admittedly a small part, of the light from fluorescent tubes. UV-A and -B are given out by sun lamps which is why the appropriate dark glasses should always be used. The near infra-red (infra-red A) is emitted by arc lamps and even by electric fires, while the far infra-reds (infra-reds B and C) are given out by furnaces.

For virtually all of history the sun has been by far the most powerful light source humans have had to deal with. It is so powerful that to gaze directly at it is to court visual disaster. The tale from African/Jamaican mythology about Anansi, outlined earlier in this chapter, paints a reasonably accurate picture of the visual effects of inadvertent sun-watching. Sometimes sun-watching is not inadvertent: numerous young Americans in the 1960s and 1970s tried to avoid being called up for the Vietnam War by sun-gazing and thus burning their retinas.

However, the sun is no longer the most powerful light source on earth because now, through advances in technology, we have laser light. All sorts of lasers, of hugely different wavelengths, are used in our modern-day environment. The lasers used for changing the shape of the cornea (see chapter 3) are in the ultraviolet; large industrial lasers like the carbon dioxide laser emit in the far infra-red; while many lasers emit coherent light in the visible spectrum and are seen as various colours appropriate to their wavelength.

Often we are not aware of how powerful and how potentially dangerous lasers can be. Helium/neon lasers emit in the visible range and they give out a very bright red light. These lasers can be made relatively small and were adapted for use as lecture-room pointers. The first one I ever used cost several hundred pounds; it was about two foot long and had to be held in both hands. The lasers decreased in size and cost so that now they are often smaller than a pen and can be obtained for a few pounds.

The light energy of one of these small lasers is thought by experts to be unlikely to produce permanent retinal damage from casual exposure, but their ability to dazzle, disorientate and cause temporary visual disturbance is considerable. In the wrong hands, they are a weapon in every sense of the word and an extremely inexpensive one at that. The laser shown in Figure 6.2 is on a key ring and, although only inches long, can put a dazzling red dot on to the wall of a house more than 100 metres away. Similar 'pointers' have been shone into the eyes of pilots landing aircraft, school bus drivers, train drivers and so on. The potential for serious accidents through misuse of these laser pointers is alarming to say the least.

Devices that emit light beyond the visible range, and laser power, have brought considerable benefits to the way we live, but also they bring with them extra visual hazards of which we need to be aware. Respect for these forms of light emission and use of appropriate safety glasses and goggles are crucial. There may be visual effects, however, that develop over long periods of exposure to lower levels of both visible light and light outside the visual range. Whether such forms of exposure are damaging to the eyes is a matter of controversy, but if the hazard is real, far larger numbers of people will be at risk.

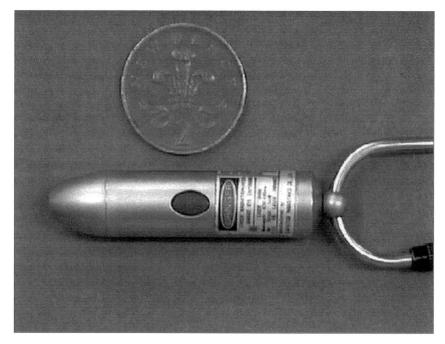

Figure 6.2   This little pen was given as a gift to a friend of mine. It can throw a laser beam
of red light more than 100 metres!

Much of the ultraviolet in sunlight that gets into the eyes is absorbed by
the cornea, and as we get older more short wavelength visible light also is
taken up by this tissue. As mentioned earlier, we have defences that limit
the amount of short wavelength light that reaches our eyes. However, an
expanse of snow defeats our defence mechanisms by reflecting light up at
our eyes. Painful corneal problems resulting from this reflected light can
be experienced by the unwary skier, and those living in areas of snow and
high levels of natural light are at risk of developing corneal opacities. How
do these obscure problems affect us? The argument is that far more reflected
light reaches our eyes now than in times past, particularly if we live in
towns. Pavements and concrete buildings are not as efficient at reflecting
light as is snow, but they are still very effective.

Light certainly seems to contribute to cataract formation because studies
show that the closer a person lives to the equator, the higher is their risk
of suffering a cataract. In addition, evidence from warm countries shows
that this risk is also increased the longer a person stays in the sun each
day. One of the culprits accelerating cataract formation would seem to be
UV-A. Age-related macular degeneration (see chapter 4) is also thought by
some to be brought on more rapidly by over-exposure to light. It is the
case that the cones, which dominate the macular region of the eye (where

there is the highest level of light exposure), are far less able to repair themselves than the rods. Although scientists do not understand very well the true effects of sunlight on the eyes, it would seem to make sense to wear good quality sunglasses when you are out in the sunshine.

Controversy exists over the possible damaging effects to the eye of long-term exposure to computer monitors. As yet there is no evidence to show clearly that ocular problems are brought on by looking at computer screens. In fact the fluorescent lighting found in many offices may be of more concern. They give out low levels of UV-A and a great deal of short wavelength visible light (blue light). Again it is not known what effect, if any, they have on the human eye, but when laboratory animals have had prolonged exposure to fluorescent light their retinal photoreceptors have been damaged. The animals investigated have in the main been those species that are normally active at night, so their eyes would be particularly vulnerable. However, it is a point made by Professor J. Marshall, a light and laser expert, that we are the first generations in which significant numbers work in office and industrial environments of fluorescent light tubes, have much of our indoor sport and recreation in a similar lighting environment (plus laser and strobed light as well at shows and nightclubs), and perhaps go home to some fluorescent lighting. We are running our own light damage experiment on ourselves, and here's hoping we get away with it!

FACTS AND OLD WIVES' TALES

✧ That rays and powers of various sorts come from the eyes is a widely held belief in many societies. One example is shown by the central African sculptures of gods that are usually made with the gods' eyes opened only to slits. If the eyes were fully open, all the powers and evils of the other world could emanate from them.

✧ It is said by sociologists that if a person says one thing with verbal language and another with body language, almost invariably we trust the body language first. If your partner has a faraway look, but says, 'No, I am not bored', which statement would you believe?

✧ On the other hand, according to my wife, I have little skill in body language. I continually read such statements as 'Of course it's OK if you don't come to the supermarket with me', and 'We don't have to leave the party early' at face value. It is said that schizophrenics, depressives and alcoholics, among many others, have poor body and social language skills. Perhaps that is why they are always there, with me, at the tail end of parties.

✧ 'I was dreaming all night.' This cannot be true because dreams take up only about one-sixth of sleep time. Dream time always seems far longer than it really is.

✧ Computer monitors are blamed for causing all sorts of eye problems, but, as yet, there is little proof that they cause any visual harm.

Chapter 7

All-seeing eye
Visual impairment now and in the future

In this final chapter I will try to deal with some aspects of the world-wide problem of visual impairment. In the west we have an ageing population and many eye problems are associated with old age. In the developing world, the population is ever increasing, and there are just too many people for the resources available. What should be done, what is being done, what isn't being done and what can't be done?

Finally I will address the most difficult part of this book, an attempt to look into the future and at the advances that might be made to combat the rising tide of visual problems. What will the future hold for all of us?

WORLD BLINDNESS

No one knows how many blind and severely visually impaired people there are in the world, but without doubt it is a very large number. Conservative estimates from World Health Organization sources suggest figures of around 50 million, which is not much less than the whole population of the UK.

What are the main causes of blindness? (Figure 7.1)

The top three are:

1. Cataract   20.0 million
2. Glaucoma   8.0 million
3. Trachoma   7.5 million

These are huge numbers in anyone's terms, but blindness and visual impairment are on the increase throughout the world and indeed these figures may well be very conservative. Much depends on the definition of blindness, and if we include those with a severe visual disability, a figure of 200 million would not be absurd and that equates to the population of western Europe or the USA. Increase in visual impairment is a problem shared by both the developed and the developing worlds. However, although the problem may be shared, the causes are different.

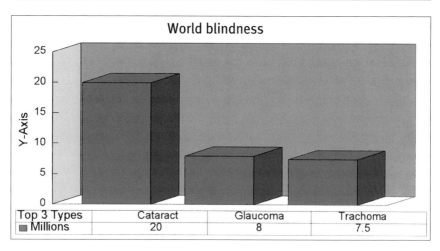

Figure 7.1   The three top causes of blindness in the world.

Failed eyes

To those involved in eye care, loss of sight and blindness are a failure. Why are there failures? Can we generalize? If we do, we might end up with the following list:

1. *Failure because, as yet, there is no cure for the eye disease.* The eye doctors can neither reverse the eye disease nor can they stop it. The doctor can only hope that science and medical advances can come up with something in the future, hopefully the near future. Diseases such as retinitis pigmentosa and most ARMD are examples (see chapter 4 for more on these diseases).

2. *Failure of the treatment used to combat the eye complaint.* The patient comes to the doctor but, despite appropriate medical or surgical treatment, vision is lost. Unfortunately success can never be guaranteed; medical treatments and operations are not successful for all, even when the most advanced procedures are available. In a world of uneven medical resources, in some regions the quality of care is unfortunately less than ideal.

3. *Failure to treat the disease in the first place.* Either because of, for example, fear of doctors or lack of finance, the patient doesn't visit the doctor, or, as is the case far too often in some parts of the world, there is no eye doctor to visit. The fact that cataract, a surgically treatable condition (see chapter 4), is by far the main cause of blindness in the world is a sad and alarming proof of the significance of this type of failure.

4. *Failure to prevent the disease from being part of the community.* There

are eye diseases that just should not be part of our lives. Large numbers of children go blind because of starvation and a lack of vitamin A (see chapter 4).

POOR BLIND EYES

In the developing world the incidence of severe visual impairment is far greater than in the developed world. This is due to shortages in health care in general, the presence of blinding diseases which are not found in the developed world and sometimes a reluctance to visit the eye doctor until the problem is too advanced for effective treatment. Among the causes of 'failure' listed above, people in the developed world have the first and second as their main worries, whereas in the developing world they are all concerns.

Shortages

In developing countries, blindness is largely a result of poor public health, a population boom, poverty and, most of all, a severe shortage of eye doctors in the right places and with the correct training. In some areas of Africa there is only one ophthalmologist for every million people, compared with the wealthy USA where there is one ophthalmologist for less than twenty thousand people or Germany where the ratio is as good or even better. As well as a lack of eye doctors, there is also an almost complete absence of the infrastructure of health professionals that is expected in developed countries, optometrists, orthoptists, specialist nurses and so on.

Cataract problems

Cataract deserves special mention. This is a major predicament everywhere in the world and even in the most developed countries there are people who are profoundly visually handicapped with cataract. However, there are also 'hot spots' where the incidence of cataract is unusually high and the age of onset is much younger than would normally be expected for an 'ageing' disease. The hottest spot of all is India, which has the highest incidence of cataract in the world. In India there is a never-ending battle against the blindness that cataract brings, a battle in which the Indian medical professions have come up with ingenious methods for combating it. One of these methods is the establishment of cataract camps where surgery is performed on an assembly line basis by doctors and specially trained surgical assistants.

The doctors operate rapidly and efficiently with amazing skill, but still the numbers increase. Anywhere between 20 and 200 operations per day will be undertaken per surgeon, compared with the 3 to 8 per day that would be performed in a UK eye hospital. A friend and colleague of mine often talked about his first introduction to surgery as an Indian ophthalmologist, and that was in a rusty old van which toured about the countryside and served as both consulting room and a store for hospital equipment. The vans go round from village to village, set up a temporary operating theatre in the van or a nearby centre and do as many operations as possible before going on to the next village. There are always too many villages.

The unpalatable truth is that, despite the efforts of so many dedicated professionals, the number of cataract operations performed each year does not come close to the number of people becoming disabled over the same period, so the numbers of blind people in India steadily increase. India is not the only country in this predicament; it is the current trend in the developing world. It is not just a matter of insufficient cataract surgery to cover a country's needs. Surgery can be performed quite successfully, but after a while the patient is effectively blind. In the 1990s the cataract operation of choice in many developing countries (because of training, cost and speed of operating) is one following which the patient will be required to wear thick glasses in order to see properly. If the glasses are lost or broken, the patient more than likely will not be able to obtain or afford a replacement pair.

Without glasses the patients will be little better off than they were before their cataract operations. As any lost property person will tell you, glasses frequently go astray and there are mountains of them lost each year. For example, if villagers are working in wet rice fields, when their glasses fall off they will be submerged in a foot of water and mud and easily lost. It has been estimated that the cost of a cataract operation in some parts of the world is as little as £10–15 so fitting intraocular lenses (see chapter 4) as an alternative to wearing cataract glasses has not been, up until recently, a practical financial proposition for many developing countries. However, as the price of intraocular lenses has fallen, more cataract operations fitting this type of lens have been performed. The problem is that a cataract operation with intraocular lens fitment is a much slower operation, so fewer patients can be treated each day.

Other problems

Trachoma, the third most common blinding eye disease, would not exist at all, or at least would be a minor issue, if public health was all that it might be in the countries where the infection is rife (the fourth type of failure in the earlier list). This is a clear case of blindness that could be prevented if only sanitation was better and eyes were not continually infected and reinfected with the chlamydia bugs that provoke the corneal scarring.

If trachoma was the only example of preventable visual impairment, it would be bad enough, but large numbers of children go blind because of insufficient vitamin A in their meagre diet. A few greens, some oil or a vitamin supplement would make all the difference; the problem is not just poverty but education as well. Large numbers of Africans and Latin Americans suffer from river blindness, their loss of sight and blindness, being due to the ravages of a parasitic worm. The worms would not be there if the biting flies that carry them were either eradicated or controlled. Many attempts at eradication have been undertaken, but as yet the flies still thrive.

Glaucoma is of course evident all over the world, but in Africa primary open angle glaucoma (the most common form there as it is in Europe and the USA) has a far earlier onset (it can be found in people in their twenties) and is more severe. Glaucoma can be treated with drops, but the drops have to be taken every day, often several times a day, for life. In the rural areas of many African countries, and in many other regions around the world, such an option is not practical. For one thing, there are not the resources; in addition, the patients may well not take the drops, and often their home conditions are such that, even with the normal preservatives present, the drops deteriorate or, even worse, become dirty and infected. Surgery is considered by many authorities as the only option to combat visual loss, but then there is the further problem of having insufficient eye doctors on hand to do the specialized operations. It is a sad irony also that people of African and Asian origin have a far poorer success rate than Europeans with the glaucoma operation (trabeculectomy, see chapter 4). In Asia, the 'closed angle' form of glaucoma is more prevalent. There, as in Africa, the glaucoma is often very advanced before the patient finally goes to see an eye doctor, and by that time the specialist has few options left. Glaucoma is one of the diseases in which the doctor can only save what sight is left; there is no way back.

OLD BLIND EYES

Distinctive changes take place in our eyes as we get older which make them ever more prone to common eye diseases, and there are increasing numbers in developed countries living to a ripe old age. Until 1900, the proportion of the population over 65 years of age in the UK was about 5 per cent; this had not changed much throughout the nineteenth century. The twentieth century, however, saw a period of steady increase, so that now the proportion is above 15 per cent and the climb is set to continue. Couple this with the fact that the incidence of most common eye problems, such as cataract, macular degeneration, glaucoma and late onset diabetic eye disease (see chapter 4), steadily increases among the elderly and you begin to appreciate that this problem will only become worse as people continue to live much longer.

An old 'un but a good 'un

As people age, the eye and surrounding tissues show evidence of the passage of time, and in this section it may be of value to refer back to chapter 1 for a reminder of the structure of the eye. The subtle but visible age changes don't appear so subtle when we look in the mirror in the morning. I mentioned in chapter 6 wrinkles around the eyes, so hated because they are the harbinger of old age. In addition to gaining wrinkles, the lids begin to droop a little, particularly the upper one. Sadly, the lids, despite the drooping, may not close as well as they once did, thus causing excessive surface drying during sleep. The lashes may start to bend inwards and cause irritation and pain.

The lacrimal gland tissue, which supplies tears to wash and protect the surface of the eye, and the goblet cells, which provide a thin layer of mucus as a wetting agent, shrivel and diminish so that progressively there is less fluid to wet the eye and the wetting process is not as good as it once was. Put these together with less effective lid closure, and dry eye is often the result. The elderly frequently complain of having gritty eyes, particularly in the morning when they wake up and when they are out on windy days. This is often simply due to them producing less tear fluid than they once had. Artificial tear preparations can be of some help.

It is common to notice in older people that the white of the eye has lost its sparkle as the sclera begins to yellow; the yellowing is caused by deposits of fat. Blood vessels become more obvious in the sclera and conjunctiva than they once were. A ring that looks like porcelain, and has a similar sheen, sometimes forms between the clear cornea and the yellowing sclera. The ring, called an *arcus*, is also produced by fatty deposits. Iris colour fades slightly in some people, usually remaining relatively bright around the pupil but having a bleached-out look elsewhere (Plate 17).

Many of the above are features we see in the mirror, but inside the eye there are other changes of which we are not so much aware. On the inside of the cornea the endothelial cell layer, whose job is to pump fluid out of the corneal tissue and thus keep it nice and clear (see chapters 1 and 2), loses cells steadily throughout life and these cells are not replaced. The remaining cells become larger and larger as they spread to fill in the gaps. Obviously the pumping mechanism is not as effective as it once was, but for most of us it is good enough to last our lifetime. If injury, infection or other disease comes to the cornea in old age, we are less likely to re-establish perfect clarity than previously.

In most of us eye pressure doesn't change much with age (see chapters

1, 2 and under glaucoma in chapter 4); the outflow system for aqueous drainage becomes less efficient as we get older, but this is compensated for by the changes in the ciliary processes which produce aqueous humour in the first place. The processes secrete less aqueous humour so there is less for the drain to deal with, and hence a balance is maintained. For some individuals the ageing outflow system will be more likely to become blocked and these will be at risk of glaucoma, the so-called eye pressure disease. It cannot be emphasized too often that the incidence of glaucoma does increase dramatically with age.

In middle life the ciliary muscle, which works the threads (zonules) that in turn alter the shape of the lens, loses some of its power. The lens and its surrounding elastic capsule in turn become more rigid. The slight failings in muscle and lens combine to make it far more difficult to alter the shape of the lens for close work such as reading. The accommodation process starts to let us down, resulting in the long-sightedness of old age and the inevitable trip to the optometrist. Our ocular biology tells us we are over 40 years of age, and the process is called *presbyopia* to distinguish it from the problem experienced by the long-sighted hypermetropes virtually all their lives. As might be expected, the short-sighted myopes are often able to withstand the ravages of presbyopia and do not need glasses for close work until they are very long in the tooth.

The ageing lens takes on a yellowish tinge and the central region becomes progressively more opaque. There are other types of cataract, but the age-related form predominates (see chapter 4). For all of us, if we live long enough, cataract is only a matter of time. For some, their cataracts will develop early in old age, while for others the development is much slower; however, they are an inevitable consequence of becoming old.

The vitreous gel is the shock-absorber for the retina and with this egg-white-like material filling the main cavity of the eye, it does not allow the retina to move much. The intimate contact with the retina starts to break down in those over 40 years old. Little pockets of fluid develop between the retina and the vitreous humour where contact has been lost and, in addition, aggregates of vitreous material start to float free in the cavity of the eye. When we are tired we see these as the so-called 'floaters' that drift strangely across our field of vision. The alterations in the vitreous humour are of no consequence to the vast majority of us. However, although retinal holes and retinal detachment can come at any age, the elderly are more susceptible, probably because of the loss of effectiveness of the shock-absorber.

In chapters 1 and 4 I mentioned some of the protection mechanisms that operate to keep the retina and the photoreceptors in tip-top condition throughout life. Both the rods and cones constantly renew their photoactive materials, which are rapidly damaged by wear and tear and also the effects of light itself. It is one of life's ironies that light, which is the key component of vision, also has such a corrosive effect on the visual apparatus. The dustbin for the spent photoreceptor materials is the retinal pigment epithelium, which spends a lifetime trying to digest and dispose of the waste products into the choroidal circulation.

Much more of the waste material taken up by the retinal pigment epithelium comes from rods than from cones. First of all, there are far more rods than cones in the human visual system with which the pigment epithelium has to deal, there being some 125 million rods and less than 7 million cones. Additionally, the turnover rate of rods is prodigious, with the whole outer segment stack of light-sensitive material being replaced every fortnight, whereas the cone turnover is much slower, its light-sensitive material taking up to a year to be totally replaced.

In the elderly, the rods experience little in the way of alteration, except that the outer segments with their photosensitive content are slightly longer than those found in the young eye. In the absence of chronic eye disease, the numbers of rods remain pretty constant throughout life. Cones, on the other hand, are whittled away as the years go by and there is some loss of organization of those that remain. On the whole there is not much by way of a functional consequence, but it should be pointed out that colour vision defects can be acquired in the elderly, particularly as a complication of pre-existing eye problems, for example diabetic eye disease.

Spare a thought for our over-worked retinal pigment epithelium with its lifetime's toil of processing all the spent and worn-out debris from the rods and cones. In the later years the dustbin has all the appearance of being full to the brim. Morphologists who look at the retinal pigment epithelium of the older eye are immediately struck by the abundant deposits of fatty membranous material present, which are seen very infrequently in younger eyes. It seems that the retinal pigment epithelium reaches a point in life when it takes in more photoreceptor material than it can process and then efficiently off-load.

Bruch's membrane (see chapter 1 and ARMD in chapter 4) separates the retinal pigment epithelium from the choroidal blood supply. This layer acts as a kind of filter, allowing the passage of nutrients from the blood supply to the pigment epithelium and the retina in one direction and the passage of waste products from the pigment epithelium in the other direction. Among these waste products is the degraded photoreceptor debris, but the debris does not exit easily and the passage gets worse with time. Eventually the filter begins to clog up, and bumps and lumps appear in Bruch's membrane. The bumps and lumps appear in us all and are of little consequence, except when they form in large numbers in the macular region. Elderly people whose Bruch's membranes have too many lumps and bumps concentrated in their macula regions are particularly prone to the development of ARMD.

An old but not so good 'un

In western Europe and North America most countries have reasonably similar instances of blindness and visual disablement, so as an example of the problem in the developed world I will use the UK. The source of information in the UK is the BD8 form, which has been used since the 1930s to register a person as either blind or partially sighted. The form is filled in and signed by an eye doctor before being sent to the local Social Services Department; if this form is not filled in, the visually handicapped person will miss out on some benefits. Another part of the BD8 form, which is anonymous, is sent by the doctor to the Census Office.

It is from the anonymous information sent to the Census Office (Figure 7.2) that we can obtain statistical information about the various eye conditions that are producing severe visual problems in the community. The main causes for blind registration in the UK are the following:

1. Age-related macular degeneration (ARMD)   49 per cent
2. Glaucoma   12 per cent
3. Diabetic eye disease   3 per cent
4. Cataract   3 per cent

Together these four types of eye problem account for 67 per cent of all the blindness in the UK and all four of these are particularly prevalent in the elderly. ARMD, for example, is not found in the age group 0–15 years,

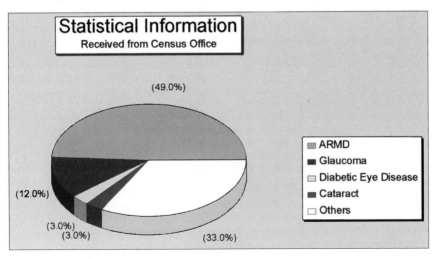

Figure 7.2 The main causes of severe visual disability in the UK based on information from the Census Office.

makes up 11 per cent of the blind in the age group 16–64 years and dominates the 65-year-olds and above by accounting for 55 per cent of the blindness of old age.

Around 14,000 people per year are certified blind in the UK and in addition 15,500 register as seriously visually handicapped (called partially sighted on the form). However, it is known that for various reasons not all people register who could do – people just do not want to admit to having a 'handicap', even if the consequence is lost benefits. No one really knows how many are not on the list, but the Royal National Institute for the Blind has estimated that for every blind person on the list there may be at least one other who is not. The figure for the partially sighted could be as bad as four not registered for every one who is. Thus if the RNIB figures are accurate, nearly 30,000 people per year go blind and 70,000 are reduced to having only partial sight. Many authorities would consider these as over-estimates of the problem, but the truth is that a more reliable figure is lacking.

What is not lacking is the very unpalatable truth that, of the blind and partially sighted people who do register, around 20 per cent have eye problems that might not have resulted in such a severe outcome had they been picked up sooner or had their treatment been more effective (both diabetic eye disease and glaucoma among others fall into this category). Also within the 20 per cent are those who are blind or partially sighted because of cataract. I have given reasons why in Africa and other parts of the developing world glaucoma treatment is not as effective as it might be, but it has to be admitted that in the UK and all other countries in the West, glaucoma remains an important cause of blindness despite the battery of available treatments. Furthermore it is extremely sobering that cataract, although by no means the blight it is in developing countries, still can be a cause of European and American blindness.

FUTURE EYES

After ploughing your way through this book and particularly this chapter, which carries with it an inevitable air of doom and gloom, a reasonable question to ask is: what does the future hold? Are we to see sometime in the future the collapse of eye care both in developed and the under-developed countries, or will there be a solution to the many problems just around the corner? What should we be doing? Are there new developments that are going to change eye care in the future?

Organization
One message of this chapter is that the vast majority of blindness in the world could be tackled by preventive measures (e.g. trachoma) or by

currently available treatments (e.g. cataract). It comes down to available resources for medicine as a whole and not just eye disease in particular, and also to such factors as public health and resource allocation. The major problem is the one we all know – that some parts of the world are far richer than others, and too many people are faced with starvation and poverty. It is in these very areas, where poverty is at its worst, that preventable and curable blindness causes most havoc.

The world problems of poverty and starvation are far too big an issue for this book, except to say that the richer countries need to give more to the poorer if the various problems (of which blindness and poor sight are only a small aspect) are ever to be brought to heel. However, as is now generally appreciated, even giving is not simple; it is complicated by politics, economics, ignorance, greed and also deciding what best to provide and where. With limited available resources, is it better for the governmental and private agencies of the West to send money or supplies, provide medicines, build hospitals or train specialists? In truth all of these are necessary, but training must have a high priority.

Training support provided to the developing world by richer countries is not just a good thing, but vital for the health of the world. Eye health in particular needs precise skills and considerable knowledge; how should support for training be provided? A simple question to which there should be a simple answer, but there is not. Britain, as with most of the richer countries in western Europe, North America and elsewhere that have sophisticated local training schemes, attracts regulated numbers of oversees doctors to its training programmes.

These doctors may be in the country for general ophthalmic eye training, for more specialized fellowship training in a specific aspect of eye care or to conduct some research. My own eye unit is fairly typical and currently we have doctors from Egypt, India, Pakistan, Jamaica, Turkey, Romania, Mauritius and Brazil who will spend anything from one to eight years in training at various centres, including our own. Training these overseas eye doctors alongside British eye doctors in this way seems ideal, but there are some problems with this type of approach which are not immediately obvious.

First of all, the cost of the training is not always borne by Britain, and the home country may have to pay all or make a substantial contribution to the expenses. The trainees are chosen for their ability, and it is irrelevant to their selection whether or not their country of origin has a particular need for eye doctors. The doctors are trained in the latest techniques needed to combat the eye problems of the western world (as required for British doctors) and during their training they will not see, for example, trachoma or river blindness and the other eye diseases that plague the developing countries. Further, the clinical approach and operating procedures in Britain and at home, because of social and economic reasons, may be entirely different. For instance, the cataract operation of choice in Britain may not be so useful in parts of the developing world where speed of operating and lack of resources come into play.

The fundamental problem is that the UK trains too few eye doctors from developing countries and those that are trained are trained too slowly. Even more of a problem is the fact that the British-trained eye doctors have skills appropriate to the rich minority in their home country who live in cities, but not to the poor rural populations where most of the visually handicapped are to be found. As a consequence, many of the doctors equipped with an expensive training from the developed world tend to work where they can treat what they have become used to managing, the older (richer) patients rather than the masses in the over-stretched eye camps. There is also the substantial loss to the developing world of those eye doctors who after training stay on in the developed world.

There are in Britain community-based training schemes for eye doctors and health professionals which are more in tune with the world of the eye camp. They are for obvious reasons very strong on theory but, at least until the trainees get home, not on practice. A lot of stress should be placed on training being focused in the home country and to that end there are very high-profile schemes such as *Orbis*. This is an American DC–10 aircraft which has been equipped with an eye operating theatre and all the modern facilities. The plane flies into various countries with surgical teams and teachers, so that local doctors and nurses can be given training and experience in surgical techniques. A Russian ship has done a similar job travelling the world and is a large floating eye hospital. These organizations do, however, appear to be as much concerned with propaganda as they are with saving sight, flag-waving for the cleverness of the West or Russia without making more than a slight dent in the problems of blindness and visual impairment in the developing world. To be fair, these organizations are now far more aware of this criticism than they once were: Orbis is establishing fixed training centres in various parts of the world and is addressing the important nutritional and preventable eye diseases it once ignored.

I am of the opinion that large numbers of formal and informal training associations should be established between eye hospitals in the developed and the developing countries. Such associations serve as a conduit whereby training can be tailored to what is needed. A valuable opportunity is offered to eye doctors from both places to share their expertise. In addition, long-term collaborative research using collective skills and experience and focused on the major sight-threatening problems of the developing world can then be undertaken. This type of 'twinning' is not new: Moorfields

Eye Hospital in London has a long-standing association with, among others, St John's of Jerusalem, the St Paul's Eye Unit in Liverpool has close contacts in Kenya, and eye institutes in the USA traditionally have established training programmes with those in Central and South America. I would like to see far more financial and political encouragement for close contact between departments, institutes and various organizations, so that together the ever-mounting problems of eye care can be tackled in an efficient and effective manner.

Research and development

If organization and finance are a problem as regards visual impairment in the developing world, then it is more emphasis on research and development that is needed in the West. We need to be able to treat diseases like ARMD that at present are not treated at all well, and also to treat diseases like glaucoma that at present are treated reasonably well but need even more effective treatments. If we consider all the various eye problems covered in this book (see chapter 4), they can basically be divided into two groups according to the type of visual loss: direct and indirect.

Direct visual loss occurs as a result of diseases and conditions that affect the retina, the optic nerve or the visual centres in the brain; these would include, for example, glaucoma, ARMD and retinitis pigmentosa. On the whole, eye doctors are not too successful with these. There is as yet no treatment for retinitis pigmentosa (produced by the loss of photoreceptors), in very few patients is ARMD brought under control (loss of the macula) and glaucoma (loss of the fibres that take the visual information from the retina to the brain) at best can be halted, but what is lost cannot be replaced. Perhaps only in cases of simple retinal detachment (where the photoreceptors split away from the retinal pigment epithelium) is the patient delighted with the visual improvement the eye doctor can bring when the retina is reattached.

Indirect visual loss occurs when, in theory at least, the retina is normal but not enough light reaches it to allow useful vision. Basically the clear parts of the eye become cloudy, as occurs when there is blood in the vitreous humour, cataract of the lens, cells in the anterior chamber, or corneal opacity. It is in treatment of these types of complaint that there can be a dramatic return of vision. Spectacular improvement of sight after a cataract operation is extremely gratifying, and thankfully commonplace, and when a clear corneal graft replaces opaque diseased cornea then a function may well be restored to the eye.

Research may provide improvements in treatment for those eye problems that have an indirect effect on vision and they would be very welcome. It should be pointed out that attempts to develop a medical preventive treatment for cataract have proved singularly unsuccessful to date, but work goes on in the search for that elusive breakthrough. Cataract surgery, on the other hand, has evolved tremendously in the past few years, with developments occurring at a bewildering speed. The quality of life for patients who have had cataract operations will steadily improve over the next decade or so.

Research and development needs to address and is addressing those illnesses in which the loss of vision is directly linked to the visual network itself. For ARMD it is surgical rather than medical developments that are showing the most promise. Many new ideas and procedures are being developed, but as yet none are in general use. Laser treatment of the 'wet' form of ARMD (see chapter 4) is undergoing further refinement. In addition, a procedure is being evaluated whereby a light-sensitive chemical is selectively absorbed by the vascular scar close to the macula (the scar causes much of the visual disturbance). When the scar is filled with the chemical, it withers away on exposure to an accurately aimed beam of light. The treatment, called photodynamic therapy or PDT (see also chapter 4), has completed successful trials, which indicate that PDT will be a useful treatment for at least some, although by no means all, patients with the wet form of ARMD.

In ARMD the support tissue beneath the macula is disorganized and degenerate, vascular scars form and the retinal pigment epithelium in that region is worn out. A variety of new operations are being developed that involve moving the macula by very precise microsurgery to a place close by where the retinal pigment epithelium isn't worn out. It sounds simple in principle, but the surgery itself isn't at all simple and has so far proved to be an operation suitable for only a few patients and conducted by a very few surgeons. Progress towards finding an easier way to move the macula from diseased tissue to a fresh site is progressing extremely rapidly. Simpler operating procedures are evolving at present in several centres and represent an exciting prospect for the near future.

The problems of ARMD have stimulated another line of research and development, and that is transplantation of retinal pigment epithelium. We know that part of the problem in ARMD is that the retinal pigment epithelium is sick and worn out, so rather than move the macula why not replace the pigment epithelium? Retinal pigment epithelial cells are grown in a special laboratory on a membrane. The surgeon lifts the macula and tidies up beneath it, then removes the worn-out epithelium, even removing the vascular scars if there are any, and inserts the new epithelium in the appropriate place. The macula is carefully put back in position and, hopefully, central vision will improve, or at least it will not deteriorate any further.

The macula is only a fraction of a millimetre in diameter, so microsurgery of this degree of precision may sound rather fanciful. However, it may surprise you to learn that eye surgery requiring this accuracy is routine and, indeed, the surgical technique for retinal epithelial transplantation is already in place. The delay in further development relates not to the transplantation procedure but to biological problems associated with the replacement epithelial cells. I suspect, however, that this technique will be available in the near future to treat some maculas, but whether or not it will be successful is another matter.

If eye doctors can transplant tiny pieces of eyes, such as corneas and maybe soon pigment epithelium, why not transplant whole eyes? Unfortunately, that is not possible now or in the near future. When an eye is removed, the optic nerve (see chapter 1) is cut, and in cutting that nerve the very thin but very long nerve fibres (which extend from all over the retina, pass in bundles down the optic nerve and extend to the brain) are also severed. It is an extremely difficult business to get nerve tissue to knit together and function properly. Even if we had the biological know-how to fix the nerve fibres, what would be left would be a surgical nightmare. There are over one million nerve fibres passing down the optic nerve, with different groups of fibres supplying different parts of the brain. Imagine the surgeon having to biologically solder all the different fibres together in the correct way, as otherwise the patient (victim?) would have very bizarre vision in the new eye.

Eye transplantation may not be just around the corner, but various kinds of 'spare part' surgery for eyes are rapidly becoming an option. Researchers have had some success in transplanting segments of retina from one eye to another. These segments retain a degree of visual function and, even though the results are not terribly impressive, it does show that some form of partial retinal replacement for patients with a defunct retina may be possible in the future. Eye tissue and cell transplantations to treat various conditions including retinitis pigmentosa, glaucoma, dry eye and a host of others are being researched (unfortunately with no certainty of a positive outcome).

Transplantation of corneal cells onto an artificial cornea might be a practical alternative to transplanting a whole donor cornea as is done at present. Around the world there is never enough fresh cornea for all the patients who need corneal transplants. In Britain the problem is not as bad as elsewhere, mostly because of the tireless activities of the National Eye Banking Service, but there is no room for complacency. Transplantations of scleral tissue and of conjunctiva are now reasonably well-established treatments for some conditions.

The next few years may well be the era of spare part surgery for eyes, but I also believe this will be the time of 'preventive' and 'rejuvenation' therapy for eyes. The first type of treatment protects cells or tissue from the ravages of a disease, while the second tries to restore what has been lost.

Many of the cells within the eye never replace themselves. The eye is related to the brain and they have this feature in common. The retina is full of nerve cells which cannot replace themselves, so when a disease strikes, the very best that can be done is to stop or slow down the visual deterioration, and too often just to watch as the loss of vision continues unabated. As has been said before, at present we do not do as well as we would like in treating diseases with a direct effect on the retina and other parts of the visual pathway.

The mechanisms by which the nerve fibres of the retina and brain protect themselves from harm are just beginning to be understood, and also scientists have started to identify as yet just a few of the components of the chemical soup that surrounds each nerve fibre, components that are also involved in keeping the nerve fibres healthy. Some protect from damage the fibres that lead from the retina to the optic nerve, while others help the photoreceptors, the rods and cones, regrow lost segments so that they can become functional once again. Scientists in universities, hospitals and drugs companies currently are very active in the research and development of drugs that either directly protect the retinal nerve tissue from harm or stimulate the release of the natural defensive agents by the eye tissues. This type of treatment is called *neuroprotection* or *retinoprotection*.

It is likely that neuroprotective drugs would help to look after the retina during and immediately after retinal detachment. They might also be of value in treating the retinal and macular degenerative diseases by slowing the pathological processes down or at least making the visual elements less susceptible to damage. It seems, however, that the eye disease that will get most of the initial attention is glaucoma. In chapter 4 it was noted that glaucoma patients have high pressure in their eyes and this high pressure damages and kills the nerve fibres that take the messages from the retina to the brain. Treatment at present is varied, but whether medical or surgical the aim is to lower eye pressure until it is no longer harmful. Neuroprotection and eye pressure treatment would be combined to protect the retina and optic nerve even more effectively from the ravages of glaucoma.

Gene therapy also can be considered in its own way a preventive therapy. This controversial type of treatment has stayed for the most part on the drawing board, and some people at least hope it will remain there. In many diseases, including some affecting the eye, part of the genetic information carried by specific cells either is not working or is working to the tissue's disadvantage. Genetic engineering aims to introduce new genetic information into the target cells so that they behave 'better' and thus the progress of the disease can be controlled.

Some people, including some very vociferous scientists, think that gene therapy is dangerous tinkering with the essence of life; others, equally voluble, think that it is the way ahead for medical treatment in the future. It will certainly be the case that the eye will figure prominently in the development of gene therapy techniques. This is partly because some of the major retinal and corneal degenerative diseases may benefit from this type of technological development, but also because factors such as the size and shape of the eye make it particularly amenable (if the treatment will work at all, it should work in the eye).

I am reasonably confident that a host of new treatments will be available in the next few years that will 'prevent' eye diseases from getting worse, and they will be even more effective than those currently in use. But what about treatments that will 'rejuvenate' eye tissue, thus bringing back that which has been lost in the progress of an eye complaint? Rejuvenation therapy is in many ways the Holy Grail of eye treatment, or it may be the equivalent of the alchemist's conversion of base metal into gold – ever hoped for but never achieved. All eye doctors have patients whose vision has been stopped from deteriorating further but who have lost a great deal sight already that can't be restored. It must be intensely frustrating to have to say to a patient, 'I'm sorry but that is the best vision you are going to get.'

Many eye problems, particularly those of old age, arise because the eye has too few of a given type of cell. The cells are lost but are not replaced. In glaucoma, for example, pressure in the eye increases because the outflow system becomes blocked owing to there being insufficient cells remaining to keep it functional. Also in glaucoma, the retina does not function well because there are too few nerve fibres to take the retinal signals to the brain. The cornea becomes cloudy in various diseases for a number of reasons, but a major one is that the corneal endothelial cells (see chapter 1) are lost and are not replaced. They line the inside of the cornea and pump water out of the cornea to keep it transparent; if there are too few of them, the cornea becomes cloudy. Dry eye occurs, partly because there is less tear fluid, but also because there are fewer goblet cells in the conjunctiva (chapter 1). This means there is less mucus available and the tear film breaks up too quickly. These are but a few examples of eye problems that might benefit from rejuvenation therapy.

Is rejuvenation therapy a pipe dream? In some circumstances the answer is 'Yes, for the moment', but in others there is a real chance that an effective therapy can be developed. There are cell systems in the eye that never divide under any circumstances, such as the retinal nerve fibres of the retina lost in glaucoma. On the other hand, cells such as the corneal endothelial cells, the meshwork cells of the outflow system, and the retinal pigment epithelium do divide, but they are strongly inhibited from so doing by individual chemical inhibitors within each of the cells. The search is now on to find these inhibitors and also to find ways of overcoming their effects. Once that is achieved, rejuvenation therapy to treat some forms of corneal disease, high eye pressure in glaucoma, dry eye and even some retinal degenerations will blossom.

We have examined biological vision and what might happen in the future, but there is also artificial vision to consider. Anyone who watches *Star Trek: the Next Generation* on TV will know of a character called Jordi Laforge, who is biologically blind, but actually sees far better than his colleagues on the *Enterprise* because of a miracle visor that gives him artificial sight. How close are we in the twenty-first century to that? Unfortunately nowhere near, but there are a number of systems in the pipeline, and two are worth mentioning. The first I will call, for convenience, 'sight bypassing the eye', whereas the second is 'sight using the eye'. A worry is that we have been here before.

Work undertaken in the USA and Europe (some of it at the University of London) in the early 1970s indicated that it might be possible to have an artificial, limited form of vision for the blind. The trouble was that, although the theory was reasonably sound, the equipment wasn't and the result was many disappointed people who had believed that a visual revolution was just around the corner. Research of this type fell into disrepute, and I was brought up, perhaps unfairly, to treat research into artificial vision with a great deal of scepticism. It is now more than 25 years since the first claims for artificial vision were made. Are there ever going to be useful, artificial vision systems for the blind and partially sighted and, if so, when? I don't know when – the current developments are still too crude and there are biological problems to solve – but this time artificial vision does seem to be on the way, hopefully sooner rather than later.

Eye bypass

If you look back at previous chapters (chapter 2 and 6 in particular), you will be reminded that we do not see with our eyes but with our brains. The eye takes light and turns it into electrical impulses, which go to the visual cortex of the brain by way of the optic nerve. In the visual cortex and other brain centres, electrical information is processed into sight as we know it. Dr Dobelle and an international group of colleagues bypass the blind eye with an electrical set-up of their own. They have developed a system based on a digital video camera in a pair of glasses, a computer (backpack) and an electronic gizmo at the back of the head. The camera's information bypasses the eye and is translated by the computer, which in turn sends its information to the gizmo and from here to the brain. This is not a system by which a blind person can really 'see'. The electrical stimulation through the gizmo's multiple electrodes causes flashes of light in the brain: the blind person does not see a wall in front, but appreciates a series of dots and flashes that he or she can be trained to 'recognize' as a wall and so on.

Much development has continued with the camera and the computer over the years, but there are worries about the gizmo, which actually fits into the head. This needs to be fitted by a neurosurgeon, and there are concerns about infection and blood clots. In the long term, could all this electrical stimulation cause brain problems? Epilepsy had been suggested as an outcome. We just don't know because much of the research has gone on behind the closed doors of commercialism. The system is limited really by the number of electrodes in the gizmo needed to form a pattern. These instruments will become better and more 'user friendly' in the very near future, but they will cost a large amount of money. An initial outlay of $50,000–100,000 is suggested, and continuous upgrades will be needed. No wonder big firms are interested!

The eye route

This system is being developed in Europe and in the USA, and at the moment the Americans appear to be way out in front. The system also works via a digital camera fitted to glasses. The camera information does not go directly to the brain, but feeds its digital visual signal to a wafer-thin diode that has been surgically implanted into the retina of the eye itself. The information from the diode then passes to the visual cortex of the brain by means of the body's own relay system – the nerve fibres of the retina and optic nerve. The visual array on the diode is a limiting factor: the very first patients have had an array of only 64 or so visual receptors to replace a biological system that has millions. I understand that the first patient had his diode system fitted for 30 minutes and could make out the letter H; then the system was removed for ethical reasons.

The research group is very high powered and has equally high expectations, but it has a long way to go to develop a useful visual system and to overcome problems, not the least of which is the rejection of the diode by the delicate retina. In the long run, the visual results may well be better with this than with the previous eye bypass system, but it will not work for all forms of blindness and visual limitation because the patient needs to still have a 'live' retina. This research group has influential backers ranging from politicians to pop stars. The blind singer Stevie Wonder (see chapter 5) is heavily involved with these scientists.

EYE KNOW

The eye is an amazing organ that provides the dominant sense of our species. Its complexity is such that Darwin even began to doubt his evolutionary theory when he thought about how such a thing could have arisen. I have outlined the structure and function of the eye, charted the rise of ocular health care, described some of the many ways in which the health of the eye goes wrong, discussed the eye problems of some well-known people of past and present, examined the impact of visual dominance on everything from society to religion, and finally considered the huge problem for the underdeveloped and the developed worlds of increasing visual problems and even blindness.

Professor Robert Weale, in his book *The Ageing Eye*, predicted that many of the working parts of the eye have a maximum working life of 120 years. As has been stated, ours is an ageing population in which substantial numbers of people do not receive anything like 120 years of normal function from, for example, their outflow system (high eye pressure and glaucoma), their lens (opacities and cataract) and their macula (loss of central vision through ARMD).

In this chapter, I have attempted some crystal ball gazing and made some predictions (always dangerous) regarding how science and medicine may well develop some exciting new advances that will give more and more people better quality of sight in their old age. The challenge for us in the developed world is to reach ever closer to a 120-year functional lifespan for all the different working parts of the eye, so that all of us can experience high-quality vision throughout our lifetime. The challenge also, particularly in the developing world, is to provide ocular health care to everyone who needs it, so that no one suffers blindness from preventable and treatable disease. 'War on want' should include 'war for sight'.

FACTS AND OLD WIVES' TALES

✧ Modern suture thread for putting stitches in the eye is so fine that it measures half the diameter of a human hair.

✧ In an eye operation it is never the case that the eye is removed and then put back in at the end. I can remember my granny telling everyone after her cataracts were treated that the surgeon had taken her eye so far out it rested on her cheek. This brought her a great deal of attention, but it wasn't true then and still isn't.

Glossary

ACANTHAMOEBA — an organism that lives in the water supply and can cause severe corneal infection in contact lens wearers who sterilize their lenses incorrectly.

ACCOMMODATION — the mechanism by which the lens in the eye changes shape as an object comes closer so that its image remains sharp on the retina.

AGE-RELATED MACULAR DEGENERATION (AMD OR ARMD) — a degenerative disease of the macula.

ALLERGIC CONJUNCTIVITIS — conjunctivitis caused by an immune response to a material to which the eye has become sensitive.

AMBLYOPIA — a loss of visual function.

ANGIOGRAPHY — a procedure to evaluate the blood vessels and blood supply in the eye using a dye.

ANOMALOSCOPE — a specialized machine for evaluating colour vision defects.

ANTERIOR CHAMBER — the cavity in the front of the eye which is filled with aqueous humour.

AQUEOUS HUMOUR — the fluid that circulates in the chambers at the front of the eye and is responsible for eye pressure.

ARCUS — a ring of fat deposits which collects around the edge of the cornea in the elderly.

ASTIGMATISM — blurring of vision produced by irregularities in the cornea or lens.

ASTROCYTE — a type of cell found in the brain, nerves and eye; also called a *glia*.

BASEMENT MEMBRANE — a substance on which cells rest.

BATES THERAPIST — an alternative medicine practitioner who considers that eye defects can be treated by exercises.

BIFOCAL LENSES — lenses combining a distance lens and a reading lens.

BINOCULAR VISION — a fused image formed by the combination of the images from the two eyes, each of which is slightly different.

BIPOLAR CELL — a type of nerve in the retina.

BLACKFLY — a biting fly that lives near rivers and can carry river blindness.

BLEPHARITIS – an inflammation and swelling of the eyelids.

BLIND SPOT – an area with no retina where the optic nerve enters the eye; hence there is no vision.

BLINK REFLEX – automatic and rapid closure of the lids.

BOWMAN'S MEMBRANE – part of the cornea.

BRAILLE – writing for the blind and partly sighted which is a series of bumps read by the fingers.

BRUCH'S MEMBRANE – separates the retinal pigment epithelium from the choroid.

CAPSULE – an elastic layer around the lens.

CARUNCLE – the lump at the side of the nose where the two eyelids meet.

CATARACT – a condition whereby the clear lens of the eye becomes cloudy.

CENTRAL DOMINANCE – the tendency to block out edge vision and allow central vision to dominate.

CENTRAL VISION – vision concentrated on the macula and dominated by the high resolution and colour vision associated with cones.

CEREBRAL CORTEX – the part of the brain concerned with vision and other activities.

CHIASMA – the place where the two optic nerves meet and cross on their way to the visual cortex.

CHLAMYDIA – the organism responsible for trachoma.

CHOROID – a bed of vessels that help supply blood to the retina; the choroid is part of the uvea.

CHOROIDITIS – inflammation of the choroidal vessels.

CHROMOSOME – a structure in the cell which carries genetic material.

CILIARY BODY – the tissue which houses the muscle that changes the shape of the lens in accommodation.

CILIARY MUSCLE – the muscle that changes the shape of the lens in accommodation.

CILIARY PROCESSES – lie beneath the ciliary body and produce the aqueous humour.

CIRCADIAN RHYTHM – a rhythm functioning on a 24-hour biological clock.

CLOSED ANGLE GLAUCOMA – in this form of glaucoma, the high eye pressure is caused by the iris blocking the outflow system and thus halting the drainage of aqueous humour.

COATS OF THE EYE – collectively the cornea, sclera, choroid and retina.

COLLAGEN – a structural material of the body (gristle).

COLLYRIAS – medical potions.

COLOUR BLINDNESS – the perception of fewer colours than normal.

COLOUR DEFECTIVENESS – a deficiency in colour vision that is not as severe as colour blindness.

COMPOUND EYE – the eye of insects and some other animals, which is made up of a myriad of small eyes.

CONCAVE LENS – a bevelled lens that bends rays of light outwards.

CONES – photoreceptors from the retina involved in colour vision.

CONGENITAL GLAUCOMA – glaucoma in infants and children.

CONJUNCTIVA – the thin, transparent membrane on the surface of the eyeball and the inside surface of the lid.

CONJUNCTIVITIS – an inflammation and redness of the conjunctival membrane; its thin blood vessels become swollen and cause a red eye.

CONTACT LENS – an artificial lens which fits on to the cornea of the eye and usually is made of either hard or soft plastic.

CONVERGENT SQUINT – in which the squinting eye turns inwards when the 'good' eye is looking straight ahead.

CONVEX LENS – a bowed-out lens that bends rays of light inwards.

CORNEA – the clear coat at the front of the eye.

CORTICAL CATARACT – a cataract associated with clouding away from the centre of the lens.

COTTON WOOL SPOTS – opaque spots of dead nerve tissue in the retina.

COUCHING – an old cataract operation (see *needling*).

CYCLITIS – inflammation of the tissues of the ciliary body.

DENDRITIC ULCERS – corneal ulcers produced by a viral infection.

DEPTH PERCEPTION – close co-operation between both eyes to give an estimate of distance.

DESCEMET'S MEMBRANE – a part of the cornea.

DEUTERANOPIA – colour vision defect in which green is the problem colour.

DIABETES – a disease caused by insulin deficiency and, as a consequence, too high a sugar level in the blood.

DIABETIC EYE DISEASE – a general term for a range of eye problems which can arise in the diabetic.

DILATOR MUSCLE – a muscle in the iris.

DIOPTRE – a measurement of bending of light rays.

DIPLOPIA – see *double vision*.

DISCIFORM DEGENERATION – a disease process, associated with some (wet) forms of age-related macular degeneration, which involves some of the choroidal blood vessels close to the macula.

DISCRIMINATION – the ability to tell objects apart.

DIVERGENT SQUINT – in which the squinting eye turns outward when the 'good' eye is looking straight ahead.

DOUBLE VISION – the failure to fuse the images from each eye, so that one object is seen as two.

DRY EYE – a defect in the tear film which can cause drying and damage to the surface of the eye.

EDGE VISION – side or peripheral vision, looking out of the 'corner of your eye'.

ENDOTHELIUM – a type of cell which lines the inside of structures such as blood vessels.

EPISCLERITIS – an inflammation or redness of the superficial part of the sclera.

EPITHELIUM – a type of cell which covers surfaces.

EVIL EYE – a look or stare that is supposed to bring bad luck.

EXTRAOCULAR MUSCLES – the muscles located in the orbit which move the eyes in various directions.

EYE NURSE PRACTITIONER – a nurse who specializes in aspects of eye care.

EYE PRESSURE – see *intraocular pressure.*

FIBROBLAST – the main cell of connective tissue and the cell that makes collagen.

FIELD OF VISION – central plus side vision; all that you can see.

FILARIAL WORM – the adult parasitic worm which forms skin nodules in onchocerciasis.

FLOATERS – dark objects that float across the vision, caused by the slight breakdown of the vitreous humour as we get older. They can be seen best when we are tired or when we are looking at a white surface on a bright day.

FLUORESCEIN – a yellow-green dye used by eye doctors for a number of tests.

FOVEA – a small pit in the central retina rich in cones.

GANGLION CELLS – retinal nerves whose fibres extend from the retina to the brain via the optic nerve.

GLAUCOMA – a group of diseases associated for the most part with high pressure inside the eye and always with loss of vision.

GLIA – a type of brain cell found also in the optic nerve and the retina.

GOBLET CELL – mucus-forming cell.

HYPERMETROPE – see *long sight.*

INFECTIOUS CONJUNCTIVITIS – conjunctivitis caused by an invasive organism.

INNER SEGMENT – one of the two main parts of rods and cones.

INSULIN – a hormone regulating sugar in the blood.

INTRAOCULAR LENS – literally a 'lens within the eye', this is a special plastic lens fitted at the time of cataract surgery.

INTRAOCULAR PRESSURE – the inside of the eye is at higher pressure than outside, like a football; the pressure is caused by the fluid called aqueous humour.

IRET EYE – an eye from Egyptian mythology associated with the god Ra.

IRIDECTOMY – an eye operation in which a little segment of iris is removed.

IRIDOLOGIST – an alternative medicine practitioner who considers that illness in the body can be diagnosed from patterns in the iris.

IRIS – a structure which gives the eye its colour and controls the amount of light entering.

IRIS HETEROCHROMIA – each of a person's eyes are of a different colour.

IRITIS – an inflammation of the iris.

ISHIHARA CHART – a common colour vision test based on coloured dots.

KERATITIS – an inflammation of the cornea.

KOHL – a black mixture used in ancient Egypt and even now in the Middle East as an eye protection and cosmetic.

LACRIMAL GLAND – a gland in the orbit which produces tears.

LANDOLT C TEST – a visual acuity test.

LANTERN TEST – a colour vision test based on coloured lights.

LASERS – instruments that produce a coherent beam of light of one wavelength. Lasers, which are made to produce light of different colours and power, are vital to the eye doctor for diagnosis and treatment.

LASIC – a corneal operation to correct vision.

LATENT SQUINT – the two eyes only intermittently work together.

LAZY EYE – an eye that has lost some or all of its visual function and cannot keep in step with the good eye.

LENS – a clear, crystalline structure behind the iris which focuses light on the retina.

LENS CAPSULE – a layer around the lens.

LENS CORTEX – the lens beneath the capsule.

LENS NUCLEUS – the centre of the lens.

LIMBUS – the region where the clear cornea merges into the white sclera.

LONG SIGHT – allows individuals to see well in the distance but only poorly close to.

MACULA – literally 'a spot', but this spot, containing the fovea, is where the highest concentration of cones is to be found and where most of the light is focused on the retina.

MACULOPATHY – a disease process involving the macula which can happen in diabetic eye disease.

MANIFEST SQUINT – the two eyes never work together.

MARFAN'S SYNDROME – a rare disorder which is associated with heart and eye problems. The sufferers are unusually tall and thin with extremely long fingers and toes.

MELANOCYTES – cells containing pigment.

MELANOMA – a pigmented cancer of the skin. A form of melanoma can also develop in the eye.

MESOPIC VISION – night and day vision working together.

METAPHYSICS – the philosophy of being or existing.

MICROFILARIA – the immature filarial worms (larvae) which can infect the eye and cause river blindness.

MONOCULAR VISION – vision from a single eye.

MUCUS – a slimy substance.

MÜLLER CELLS – a special type of retinal cell which helps hold the retina together.

MYOPE – see *short sight*.

NAEVI – large freckles sometimes seen on the iris.

NEEDLING – part of the process of pushing a cataractous lens out of the way, see *couching*.

NEOVASCULAR GLAUCOMA – a severe secondary glaucoma which arises in some with diabetic eye disease.

NEUROPROTECTION – a term for treatments that protect the brain and/or retinal tissue from harm and by so doing promote tissue survival.

NIGHT BLINDNESS – poor night vision, which can be due to a deficiency of vitamin A, which is needed for the action of retinal rods.

NORMAL TENSION GLAUCOMA – glaucoma which takes place without an elevated eye pressure.

NUCLEAR CATARACT – a cataract that starts at the centre of the lens and then progresses outwards.

OCULAR HYPERTENSIVES – people with high eye pressure who do not have the visual loss that occurs in glaucoma.

OCULAR MELANOMA – cancer of the eye.

OCULIST – anyone who specializes in the treatment of eyes.

ONCHOCERCIASIS – a tropical eye disease which is caused by a worm; it often leads to the eye problem known as *river blindness*.

OPHTHALMIA – an old term that was used to cover all sorts of inflammations of the eye.

OPHTHALMOLOGIST – an eye doctor.

OPHTHALMOSCOPE – an instrument for looking into the eye.

OPTIC CANAL – the passage for the optic nerve between the eye and brain.

OPTIC NERVE – the nerve which links the eye and brain.

OPTIC NERVE HEAD – where the optic nerve enters the inside of the eye; the *blind spot.*

OPTICIAN – an eye professional who gives eye tests and sells glasses or contact lenses.

OPTOMETRIST – an optician who also screens for eye disease.

ORBIS – an American DC-10 plane which is equipped as an eye surgery teaching unit and travels the world.

ORBIT – the housing for the eye.

ORTHOPTIST – a health professional concerned principally with the investigation, diagnosis and treatment of disorders of eye movement.

OUTER SEGMENT – the part of the rods and cones involved in vision.

OUTFLOW SYSTEM – the tissue which drains the fluid aqueous humour out of the eye and becomes blocked in glaucoma.

PALMING – a method used by Bates therapists for exercising eyes.

PARALYTIC SQUINT – a squint caused by damage to the extraocular muscles of the eye.

PATIENT'S CHARTER – introduced in 1992, outlining patients' rights in the UK.

PERIMETER – outer extent of the field of vision.

PHOTOPIC VISION – daylight vision.

PHOTORECEPTORS – the rods and cones of the retina.

PHOTOREFRACTIVE KERATOPLASTY (PRK) – a type of refractive surgery in which a furrow is cut in the cornea with a laser.

PINEAL GLAND – a small structure associated with the brain. In humans it produces melatonin, a hormone that helps to regulate the biological clock.

PRESBYOPIA – the long-sightedness which comes with age, and results in a need for reading glasses.

PRIMARY OPEN ANGLE GLAUCOMA – the most common form of glaucoma in Britain, which is associated with a slow increase in eye pressure; also called chronic simple glaucoma.

PROLIFERATIVE DIABETIC RETINOPATHY – a severe problem that can occur in diabetic eye disease which is associated with the growth of blood vessels and vascular scars on the surface of the retina.

PROTANOPIA – colour vision defect in which red is the problem colour.

PTERYGIUM – scar tissue induced by light, which grows across the cornea and can cause visual impairment if left untreated.

PUPIL – the hole in the iris which lets light into the inside of the eye.

RADIAL KERATOTOMY (RK) – a type of refractive surgery in which scalpel cuts are made in the cornea.

RADIOTHERAPY – treatment involving the use of radioactive materials.

RAPID EYE MOVEMENT (REM) – fast movement of the eyes beneath closed lids in sleep. REM is associated with increased brain activity while dreaming.

RED EYE – the red reflex of photography, or, an inflamed eye.

RED REFLEX – the red blood of the choroid makes the pupil look red in some flash photography; see *red eye*.

REFRACTION – the bending of rays of light by the cornea and lens to focus light on the retina.

REFRACTIVE SURGERY – surgery on the cornea to improve eyesight.

RETINA – a complex arrangement of nervous tissue at the back of the eye, concerned with the visual process.

RETINAL DETACHMENT – occurs when the retina comes away from the other coats of the eye between the photoreceptor outer segments and the retinal pigment epithelium.

RETINAL PIGMENT EPITHELIUM – a layer of retinal cells which looks after the rods and cones.

RETINITIS PIGMENTOSA – a group of retinal degenerative diseases.

RETINOBLASTOMA – a rare childhood cancer of the retina.

RETINOPROTECTION – see *neuroprotection*.

RETINOSCOPE – a machine that shines a light into the eye, through the pupil and on to the retina, and provides a measurement of the correction needed for glasses.

RHEUMATOID ARTHRITIS – an illness (inflammation) of the joints which can also affect other parts of the body like the eye.

RHODOPSIN – the visual pigment in rods.

RIVER BLINDNESS – see *onchocerciasis*.

RODS – the photoreceptors from the retina concerned with black and white vision in dim light.

SCANNING LASER OPHTHALMOSCOPE – a machine for looking at the optic nerve and retina.

SCHLEMM'S CANAL – an aqueous collecting vessel in the outflow system.

SCLERA – the white of the eye.

SCLERITIS – a severe inflammation bringing about redness of the normally white sclera.

SCOTOPIC VISION – night vision, vision in dim light.

SHORT SIGHT – allows individuals to see well up close but not into the distance.

SIDE VISION – peripheral (or edge) vision dominated by rods, looking out of the 'corner of your eye'.

SIMPLE EYE – a very basic eye which is found in various forms in snails, spiders and other animals.

SLIT LAMP – a machine used to look into the eye.

SMOOTH MUSCLE – a type of muscle, not linked to bone, which produces slow and gradual contractions.

SNELLEN CHART – an eye test to check distance vision in a visual acuity test.

SPECTACLE – a clear cover over the eye found in lizards and snakes.

SPECTACLES – lenses for both eyes linked over the bridge of the nose.

SPHINCTER MUSCLE – a muscle in the iris.

SQUINT – the eyes do not work together.

STEREOPSIS – two images fused into one.

STRABISMUS – the technical name for *squint.*

STRIPED MUSCLE – a major type of muscle which has a striped appearance and produces rapid contractions.

STROMA – a piece of connective tissue.

SUNNING – a potentially dangerous technique in Bates therapy which involves looking at the sun with the eyes closed.

SYMPATHETIC OPHTHALMITIS – after serious injury to one eye, an inflammation can arise in the other eye due to an attack on eye tissues by the body's immune system.

SYPHILIS – a sexually transmitted disease which, if improperly treated, can in its later stages produce neurological problems and blindness.

TEARS – fluid from the lacrimal gland which washes the eye.

TEAR FILM – fluid on the corneal surface.

THIRD EYE – a small number of animals have a third eye extending from the top of their head which tells night from day, but in many others a remnant remains called the pineal gland.

THIRD EYE OF SHIVA – the Hindu god Shiva is believed to have a third eye which has the power to reduce the world to ashes.

TONOMETER – an instrument used for measuring the pressure in the eye.

TOXOCARA – a worm carried by dogs, which, if taken in by people, on rare occasions can produce eye problems and even blindness.

TRABECULAR MESHWORK – part of the outflow system by which aqueous humour leaves the eye.

TRACHOMA – an infective scarring disease of the front of the eye associated with the organism *Chlamydia.*

TRIAGE NURSE – a nurse from the accident and emergency unit who works out the priority in which patients need to be seen by the doctor.

TRICHROMATIC THEORY – a theory that explains how colour vision works based on there being three types of cone.

TRITANOPIA – colour vision defect in which blue is the problem colour.

UVEA – the middle coat of the eye, which is a bed of blood vessels.

UVEITIS – inflammation of the uvea.

VARIFOCAL LENSES – graduated lenses which allow distance vision at the top and reading at the bottom, with a gradual change between.

VISUAL ACUITY – the ability of the eye to make out form, to discriminate.

VISUAL AXIS – the path of light into the eye and up to the retina.

VISUAL CORTEX – that part of the brain concerned with vision.

VISUAL FIELD – see *field of vision.*

VISUAL PERCEPTION – a brain processing mechanism whereby a 'best guess' is made of what an object may be in the absence of sufficient visual information.

VITAMIN A – a vitamin essential for vision.

VITREORETINAL SURGERY – surgery associated with difficult cases of retinal detachment, injury at the back of the eye and proliferative diabetic retinopathy.

VITREOUS CAVITY – a large cavity at the back of the eye.

VITREOUS HUMOUR – a clear jelly-like material which fills the vitreous cavity.

WEDJAT EYE – in Egyptian mythology, the eye that the god Horus lost in his battles with his uncle, Seth.

ZONULES – threads which hold the lens in place.

Further Reading

The further reading suggested is not comprehensive, but will give you more information on various topics than I have been able to offer in this book.

Chapter 1

Only for the most enthusiastic or those with related careers in mind:

Bron, A., Tripathi, R. C. and Tripathi, B. (1997), *Wolff's anatomy of the eye and orbit.* Chapman and Hall Medical, London.

Forrester, J., Dick, A., McMenamin, P. and Lee, W. (1996), *The eye. Basic sciences in practice.* W. B. Saunders, London.

Chapter 2

Again more for the enthusiast than the casually interested reader:

Adler, F. H. (1999), *Physiology of the eye.* Times Mirror, London.

Burton, R. (1970), *Animal senses.* David and Charles, Newton Abbot.

Davson, H. (1980), *Physiology of the eye.* Churchill Livingstone, Edinburgh.

Goldstein, E. B. (1996), *Sensation and perception.* Brookes/Cole Publishing, Pacific Grove.

Gregory, R. (1998), *Eye and brain. The psychology of seeing.* Oxford University Press, Oxford and Tokyo.

Gregory, R., Harris, J., Heard, P. and Rose, D. (1995), *The artful eye.* Oxford University Press, Oxford.

Zeki, S. M. (1993), *A vision of the brain.* Blackwell, Oxford.

Chapter 3

An odd mix of books that are strange bedfellows, but I hope some may be of interest:

Albert, D. A. and Edwards, D. D. (1996), *The history of ophthalmology.* Blackwell, Cambridge, MA.

Bates, W. H. (1995), *Better eyesight without glasses.* Thorsons, London.

Cobb, S. R. (1987), *Optometrist on a Scottish Hebridean island.* Vantage Press, New York.

Colton, J. and Colton, S. (1996), *Health essentials. Iridology.* Element Books, Shaftsbury.

Duke-Elder, S. (1962), *The foundations of ophthalmology.* Kimpton, London.

Okhravi, N. (1997), *Manual of primary eye care.* Butterworth Heinemann, Oxford.

Perry, J. P. and Tullo, A. B. (1995), *Care of the ophthalmic patient.* Chapman & Hall, London.

Rowe, F. (1997), *Clinical orthoptics.* Blackwell, Oxford.

Chapter 4

In addition to the books recommended for chapter 3, the following may be of interest:

Batterbury, M. and Bowling, B. (1999), *Ophthalmology – an illustrated colour text.* Churchill Livingstone, Edinburgh.

Chawla, H. B. (1993), *Ophthalmology.* Churchill Livingstone, Edinburgh.

Kennerley Banks, J. L. (1994), *Clinical ophthalmology.* Churchill Livingstone, Edinburgh.

Chapter 5

A very variable batch of reading. Some of these are fun while others are specialized, but all of them I think are interesting:

Banks, G. (1980), *Banks of England.* Arthur Barker, London.

Blunkett, D. (1995), *On a clear day.* Michael O'Mara Books, London.

Bruno, F. (1992), *The eye of the tiger.* Weidenfeld & Nicolson, London.

Charles, R. and Ritz, D. (1992), *Brother Ray. Ray Charles' own story.* Da Capo Press, New York.

Craker, C. (1992), *Get into classical music.* Bantam Books, Toronto.

Halliday, F. E. (1970), *Wordsworth and his world.* Thames & Hudson, London.

Hibbert, C. (1995), *Nelson. A personal history.* Penguin Books, London.

Keates, J. (1992), *Handel. The man and his music.* Guernsey Press, Channel Islands.

Kendall, Richard (1992), *Cézanne by himself.* BCA, London and New York.

Marmor, M. F. and Ravin, J. G. (1997), *The eye of the artist.* Mosby, St Louis.

O'Shea, J. (1993), *Music and medicine.* J. M. Dent, London.

Routledge, P. (1998), *Gordon Brown: the biography.* Simon & Schuster, London.

Taylor, D. (1985), *Frame by frame: Dennis Taylor.* Queen Anne Press, London.

Trevor-Roper, P. (1970), *The world through blunted sight.* Thames & Hudson, London.

Chapter 6

Ackerman, D. (1996), *A natural history of the senses.* Phoenix, London.

Berger, J. (1990), *Ways of seeing.* Penguin Books, London.

Binder, P. (1973), *Magic symbols of the world.* Hamlyn, London.

Cole, J. (1999), *About face.* MIT Press, Cambridge, MA and London.

Duck, S. (1986), *Human relationships.* Sage, London.

Groning, K. (1996), *Decorated skin. A world survey of body art.* Thames & Hudson, London.

Kleege, G. (1998), *Sight unseen.* Yale University Press, New Haven and London.

Kuusisto, S. (1998), *Planet of the blind.* Faber & Faber, London.

McGavin, D. D. M. (1996), 'World blindness and community eye health'. *Eye News*, vol. 3, 7–11.

McNeill, D. (2000), *The face.* Penguin Books, London.

New Larousse encyclopedia of mythology (1973). Hamlyn, London.

Packard, V. (1991), *The hidden persuaders.* Penguin, New York.

Simms, J. (no date), *A practical guide to beauty therapy.* Stanley Thornes, Cheltenham.

Weale, R. A. (1963), *The ageing eye.* Lewis and Co., London.

Chapter 7

Ask at your local library on how to get the specialised texts; there are also HMSO and WHO publications.

Evans, J. et al. (1996), 'Blindness and partial sight in England and Wales: April 1990–March 1991'. *Health Trends*, vol. 28, 5–12.

Johnson, G. J., Minassian, D. C. and Weale, R. (1998), *The epidemiology of eye disease.* Chapman and Hall, London.

Useful addresses

BATES METHOD TEACHERS
PO Box 25
Shoreham by the Sea BN43 6ZF
Tel: 0190 387 7510

BRITISH COUNCIL FOR PREVENTION OF BLINDNESS
12 Hardcourt Street
London W1H 1DS
Tel: 020 7724 3716

BRITISH ORTHOPTIC SOCIETY
Tavistock House North
Tavistock Square
London WC1H 9H
Tel: 020 7387 7992

BRITISH RETINITIS PIGMENTOSA SOCIETY
PO Box 350
Buckingham MK18 5EL
Tel: 01280 860363

BRITISH SOCIETY OF IRIDOLOGISTS
998 Wimborne Road
Bournemouth
Dorset BH9 2DE
Tel: 01202 518078

COLLEGE OF OPTOMETRISTS
42 Craven Street
London WC2N 5NG
Tel: 020 7839 6000

GUIDE DOGS FOR THE BLIND
Hillfields
Burghfield Common
Reading
Berkshire RG7 3YG
Tel: 0118 9835555

INTERNATIONAL GLAUCOMA ASSOCIATION
108c Warner Road
Camberwell,
London SE5 9HQ
Tel: 020 7737 3265

MACULAR DISEASE SOCIETY
PO Box 247
Haywards Heath RH17 5FF
Tel: 0990 143573

ROYAL COLLEGE OF OPHTHALMOLOGISTS
17 Cornwall Terrace
London NW1 4QW
Tel: 020 7935 0702

ROYAL NATIONAL INSTITUTE FOR THE BLIND (RNIB)
224 Great Portland Street
London W1N 6AA
Tel: 020 7388 1266

AUTHOR'S ADDRESS
Unit of Ophthalmology
Department of Medicine
University Clinical Departments
Duncan Building
Daulby Street
Liverpool
L69 3GA
Tel: 0151 706 4098
e-mail eye123@liverpool.ac.uk
http://www.liv.ac.uk/ophthalmology/

Index

Page numbers in **bold** type refer to figures; those preceded by an asterisk denote glossary entries